Healing Diabetes Naturally

Clinically-Tested Ayurvedic
Herbs, Formulations, Nutrients
and Foods.

Dr. Nishal Ramnunan B.A.M.S

Copyright

Copyright © 2019 by Nishal Ramnunan.
All rights reserved.
No part of this book may be reproduced or transmitted in any form or by any means without prior written permission of the author and publisher.

Liability Disclaimer

The information contained in this book is for information purposes only and is not intended to replace the services of a doctor or health-care practitioner licensed to diagnose and treat disease. Any application of the material in this book is to the readers' sole responsibility. If you have a medical condition, please consult a physician. The statements in this book have not been evaluated by the U.S. Food and Drug Administration and are not intended to diagnose, treat, cure or prevent any disease or disorder in any way or form.

Contact Info

Dr. Nishal Ramnunan B.A.M.S
Phone Number: (+1) 386-837-8873
Email: doctornishal@gmail.com
Website: www.doctornishal.com

Social Media

Facebook: www.facebook.com/doctornishal
Twitter: www.twitter.com/doctornishal
YouTube: www.youtube.com/c/NishalRamnunan

Got Questions? Need Help?

This book contains over thirty potent remedies that have demonstrated anti-diabetic effects in clinical studies. Over the years, I have used every last one of these options (as well as others that are not mentioned in this book) with+ patients/clients suffering with Diabetes and its various complications.

I have read through thousands of research papers and developed my own evidence-based protocols for managing hundreds of illnesses and have had nothing but success time and time again.

I now spend the majority of my time sharing my knowledge through seminars, workshops, lectures, videos, blogging and books. However, I absolutely love working one on one with people, and will never walk away from practicing Ayurvedic medicine as this is something that people desperately need.

The main problem that people face is finding a practitioner like me to help them with their condition(s). For this reason, I have decided to offer online consultations so that people all over the world can have access to me directly. While my schedule still gets filled up, I make sure to free up time to be available for online consultations so that people can get the help they need.

To book an Online Consultation with me, go to
www.DoctorNishal.com/consultation

Table of Contents

Introduction..6
How to Use This Book..................................8
What is Diabetes?......................................11
Role of Stress..15
Role of Heavy Metals................................17
Ayurvedic Perspective on Diabetes..........18

Evidence-Based Herbal Medicines..............23
Sage..24
Amla..27
Gymnema Sylvestre..................................31
Cinnamon..34
Vinegar...37
Salacia..39
European Ash...42
Berberine..44
Nigella Sativa...47
Stinging Nettle..50
Aloe Vera..53
Fig Leaves..56
Flax Seeds..59
Fenugreek...62
Caucasian Whortleberry............................66
Walnut Leaf...69
Jackfruit Leaf...72
Withania Coagulans..................................75
Indian Gentian..78
American Ginseng....................................81
Triphala..84

Shilajit..88
Asanadi Ghana Vati..92
Ginger..95
Garlic...98
Mehamudgara Vati...101
Phalatrikadi Kwath...105
Caper Bush Fruit Extract....................................108
Bitter Apple..111
Milk Thistle..114

Managing Diabetic Complications..............117
Retinopathy..118
Neuropathy...120
Nephropathy...124
Non-Healing Wounds...127

Diabetic Nutrition...128
Chromium..130
Vanadium...131
Benfotiamine/Thiamine......................................132
Magnesium...133
Additional Nutrients..134

Exercise, Yoga & Pranayama.......................135

Dietary Advice..140

Diabetes Type 1..147

Conclusion...153
How to Find an Ayurvedic Doctor.....................155
Bibliography..157

Introduction

My name is Dr. Nishal Ramnunan. I am an Ayurvedic doctor located in Orlando, FL. I've been trained clinically as well as classically in Ayurvedic medicine and Ayurvedic surgery. I practice evidence-based Ayurveda and natural medicine with a primary focus on chronic illnesses and lifestyle-related diseases. I have a strong passion for dealing with conditions that are difficult to treat and considered incurable.

Being in the field of alternative medicine, I tend to get a lot of patients whom suffer from complex illnesses which are often multiple in number. These patients have pretty much given up on conventional medicine and are seeking an alternative to relieve their suffering. The most common conditions among these patients are insulin resistance and Diabetes.

There is evidence linking insulin resistance to multiple illnesses including non-alcoholic fatty liver disease, poly-cystic ovary syndrome, obesity, Alzheimer's disease, heart disease, and even autoimmune conditions such as multiple sclerosis.

While the role of insulin resistance in the development of these diseases is still being investigated, it should be noted that cellular metabolic processes such as "autophagy" also appear to be inhibited by insulin – meaning that cellular detoxification may be impaired in patients with too much circulating insulin (insulin resistance).

Autophagic dysregulation and deficiencies have been seen in almost every autoimmune condition, cancer, and even neurodegenerative conditions such as Parkinson's disease.

With the potential of Diabetes and insulin resistance to destroy ones health, it should come as no surprise that I, a person who preaches preventative medicine, would choose to write a book on this topic. Based on the the fact that Diabetes is the 7th leading cause of death in the USA, I would suggest that you take this condition seriously as well.

In this book, I have discussed a wide-range of simple, clinically-tested, remedies for getting blood sugar under control and managing this condition in the most simple way with little or no side-effects.

The majority of people have no idea that simple foods and herbs found in their kitchens can effectively reduce fasting blood sugar, postprandial blood sugar, HbA1c and even assist in reducing the symptoms of Diabetic complications.

Therefore, I have compiled these remedies into one easy-to-use book that provides details on all the most common remedies together with references to clinical studies so that you are aware that whatever you use, has been tested with success in human research.

Most of my patients/clients have stated that their regular doctors express doubt towards the potential of natural medicines due to an false belief that these "medicines" have not been researched. As I have demonstrated in this book, this idea is completely untrue. In fact, there is evidence proving the efficacy of Ayurveda, nutrition and natural medicine in treating literally hundreds of diseases and symptoms.

I even have an online research library which I allow physicians to reference should they feel unconvinced about the potential of natural medicine(s).

Should your doctor have any questions or doubts, feel free to use the references at the end of this book to inform them. Literally, every study I have referenced can easily be found online.

If you have any concerns of confusion, please feel free to reach out to me directly as I am quite approachable. My contact details can be found in the beginning of this book.

I wish you good luck on your journey to better health and look forward to hearing about your success.

Sincerely,
Dr. Nishal Ramnunan B.A.M.S.

How to use this book?

1. First and foremost, I recommend using the herbs, nutrients and formulations in this book under the close supervision of a holistic physician to avoid drug interactions, adverse effects and misuse.

2. Secondly, it is important to understand the specifics of your condition – symptoms, blood sugar levels (fasting, postprandial and HbA1c), complications, medicine requirements, etc.

3. Third, you should be aware of the effects your current medicine has on your blood sugar levels.

4. If you require insulin, it is essential to use insulinotropic agents to increase endogenous insulin production – more on page 147. While using these herbs, blood sugar must be closely monitored throughout the day as standard insulin requirements may reduce.

In my experience, this can sometimes happen within the first few doses.

5. If you do not require insulin, any of the options in this book may be used. Again, blood sugar must be closely monitored as standard medicine requirements may reduce significantly from the first dose. Also, allergies & drug/herb interactions must be considered.

6. If during the course of supplementation, blood sugar levels are only decreasing slightly, then herbs/nutrients/formulations may be combined. This decision can only be made after a few weeks of being on these herbs/supplements.

Combining of herbs and formulations should be done by an experienced holistic/Ayurvedic physician.

7. Closely monitor blood sugar levels to avoid hypoglycemia (low blood sugar)

Hypoglycemia

If you experience low-blood sugar (hypoglycemia), it is essential to use **oral glucose tablets, honey or other sugar rich sources** to quickly raise blood sugar – they may not be healthy, but they may save your life. One could also consume a carbohydrate rich meal. Careful calculations must be made when treating Diabetes, that is why it must be done with a holistic doctor's guidance.

Hypoglycemia occurs when blood sugar levels are below 72mg/dl. It can result in symptoms such as:

- Tremors
- Irritability
- Accelerated heart rate
- Hunger
- Anxiety
- Sweating
- Dizziness
- Weakness
- Paleness
- Heart palpitations

Hypoglycemia can also occur at night and result in nightmares, weakness upon waking, sweating at night, and even crying during sleep.

Apart from excessive use of anti-diabetic herbs and medicines, there are other potential causes of hypoglycemia such as:

- Not eating enough
- Tumors
- Drugs
- Excessive alcohol consumption (long-term)
- Kidney disorders
- Excessive exercise or other physical exertion

In severe hypoglycemia, a patient may go into diabetic shock. This can lead to seizures, loss of consciousness and even a coma.

It is essential to make those whom are frequently around you aware of methods to help you raise your blood sugar should you find yourself in a situation unable to help yourself. Simple remedial measures like applying honey to the inside of your mouth can help to raise blood sugar if needed.

Avoid hypoglycemia with careful calculations of medicinal requirements, close monitoring of blood sugar levels, and well timed meals.

In the case of an emergency, please call 911 (USA) or whatever emergency services are available in your area.

What is Diabetes?

Diabetes Mellitus refers to a group of diseases that involve the inefficient metabolism of sugar resulting in elevated blood glucose levels. Glucose is needed to provide every cell with energy, however, excessively elevated glucose levels have detrimental effects and lead to the damage of multiple organs including the brain, kidneys, eyes, arteries, nerves and more.

The metabolism of sugar is carried out by a hormone known as "insulin". When insulin is reduced or if the cells have a reduced ability to interact with insulin, blood sugar levels become elevated.

Diabetes is generally characterized into 3 types:

- Diabetes Mellitus Type 1
- Diabetes Mellitus Type 2
- Gestational Diabetes

Diabetes Mellitus Type 2 is a chronic condition characterized by the inability of cells to interact with insulin and allow sugar to enter the cell. As a result, sugar builds up in the blood and the patient develops what is known as "Hyperglycemia". Blood sugar in these patients tends to be raised in a fasting state as well as after meals (Postprandial).

This type of Diabetes occurs during adulthood and more so in the elderly, however younger people are developing it as well, due to poor diet, lack of exercise and obesity.

Treatment usually involves the use or Hypoglycemic drugs such as Glucophage, etc.

Diabetes Mellitus Type 1 is a condition is which the hormone insulin is reduced or lacking. It is an autoimmune condition in which the immune system attacks and destroys the beta cells within the pancreas which are responsible for producing insulin, resulting in reduced insulin production. Treatment for this condition usually requires the patient to inject insulin in order to support the metabolism of sugar.

This form of Diabetes is often referred to as "Juvenile diabetes" as it commonly affects people in a younger age group.

In this book, I discuss options that improve insulin production and release. Treating this condition requires a very specific approach as autoimmune conditions have multiple factors responsible for their development – this has to be assessed and treated by a holistic physician.

Symptoms of Diabetes

- Polyuria (Excessive Urination)
- Polydipsia (Excessive Thirst)
- Polyphagia (Excessive Hunger)
- Weight Loss or Weight Gain
- Fatigue & Irritability
- Blurred Vision
- Slow Healing Wounds

How is Diabetes Diagnosed?

When fasting blood sugar is constantly raised above normal levels (<100mg/dl) over the course of several days, it indicates that the patient has impaired fasting glucose and may be Diabetic - especially if it is constantly above 126mg/dl.

When postprandial blood sugar is constantly raised above 140mg/dl is indicates impaired glucose tolerance. Above 200mg/dl indicates Diabetes.

A test known as HbA1c is used to assess the average blood sugar levels from the last three months. Results of 5.7- 6.4 indicate pre-diabetes and 6.5 or higher indicates Diabetes. To determine if the patient has Diabetes Type 1, your doctor may test for antibodies such as:

- Glutamic Acid Decarboxylase Auto-antibodies (GADA/Anti-GAD)
- Insulin Auto-antibodies (IAA)
- Insulinoma-Associated-2 Auto-antibodies (IA-2A)

- Islet Cell Cytoplasmic Auto-antibodies (ICA)
- Zinc Transporter 8 (ZnT8Ab)

*C-Peptide may be tested for as well.

<u>Gestational Diabetes</u> is a type that develops during pregnancy and like the other types, it also affects glucose metabolism. This condition is believed to increase the baby's risk for developing Diabetes at a later stage in life.

*This condition often goes away after birth.

Diabetes Type 3

As of recently, Alzheimer's disease is on the verge of being classified as Diabetes Type 3. This is because glucose metabolism issues clearly play a role in the pathogenesis of this condition. Coincidentally, several of the herbs and nutrients mentioned in this book are used for treating both Diabetes as well as Alzheimer's and/or risk factors for Alzheimer's.

Causes & Risk factors

These following put patients at risk for developing Diabetes:

Diabetes Type 1:
- Genetics
- Viral infections & other environmental factors
- Auto-antibodies
- Location

Diabetes Type 2:
- Genetics
- Poor dietary habits
- Obesity
- Sedentary lifestyle
- Age
- Hypertension & Hyperlipidemia
- Gestational Diabetes
- Poly-cystic Ovary Disease

Complications of Diabetes

- Retinopathy (Eye Damage)
- Neuropathy (Nerve Damage)
- Nephropathy (Kidney Damage)
- Heart Disease
- Gangrene
- Non-Healing Wounds
- Gastroparesis
- Alzheimer's Disease
- Hearing Impairment

Additional Info

- According to the World Health Organization, well over 300 million people currently have some form of Diabetes, and that number is rising quickly.

- In the United States, Diabetes is the 7th leading cause of death.

- More than $200 billion is spent a year for Diabetes.

- Patients with Diabetes average a medical expenditure of over $13,000/year.

- Between 5-10% of Diabetic patients have Type 1 and 90-95% have Type 2.

Role of Stress

Stress is one of three major causes of chronic disease, together with poor diet and lack of exercise. Stress results in the body behaving as though it is under attack by activating several pathways responsible for immediate energy use via the release of several hormones.

Stress can be long-term or short-term, and result from many sources such as physical injuries, excessive work, and illness as well as mental stresses such as financial, marital, or occupational difficulties. Both forms put the body into a fight-or-flight state which alters biochemistry.

If stress is long-term, it has the potential to initiate and/or contribute to the development of chronic illnesses.

During a stressful event, the hypothalamic-pituitary-adrenal (HPA) axis is stimulated – this results in the release of the stress hormone "Cortisol" and activation of the sympathetic nervous system, which goes on to increase catecholamines and interleukin-6.

- Cortisol induces insulin resistance and the accumulation of visceral fat. Both of these are precursors to Diabetes Type 2.

- Catecholamines such as Epinephrine, when in excess, increase blood glucose and both peripheral and hepatic insulin resistance.

- Interleukin-6, a cytokine (a protein produced by the immune system) plays a significant role in the developement of inflammatory illnesses and leads to insulin resistance in hepatocytes (liver cells).

Keep in mind that this description is merely that of the effect stress has on blood sugar. The complete effect of stress extends to the induction of inflammatory pathways, weight gain, hypertension, increased blood viscosity and several other factors. Stress plays a role in autoimmune disorders, metabolic disorders, weight gain, sexual disorders and heart disease. Therefore, it is imperative that stress be properly managed, relieved, or avoided.

Stress management

My recommendation is to use the following methods of stress reduction

1. Hobbies and enjoyable activities such as:
- Massage
- Listening to music as well as playing a musical instrument
- Sexual intercourse
- Watching movies or playing video games.
- Playing with a pet, etc
- Nature Walks

2. Yoga & Related Activities:
- Asanas
- Meditation
- Pranayama (Breathing exercises)

3. Adaptogenic herbs (Used under a doctor's supervision):
- These are herbs that help the body adapt to stress and reduce the levels of stress hormones. Many of them also possess anxiolytic and anti-depressant effects. Herbs such as Ashwagandha, Tulsi, Ginkgo Biloba are common adaptogens as well as Shilajit – which is generally my preference due to the fact that it is also a potent anti-diabetic substance.

Role of Heavy Metals

Recently, heavy metal toxicity has come to light as more and more evidence has linked these to the development of several chronic disorders such as Diabetes, Autism and Alzheimer's disease. While this area of study is still in its infancy, I would advise you to take this seriously as it is a known thing that we now live in a world rich in environmental toxins. Everything from our water bottles to the power cables on our clothing irons, they are all loaded with endocrine disrupting substances and carcinogens capable of contributing to the development of disease.

Heavy metals can be found in fish, vaccines, cigarettes, poorly processed foods, etc.

Heavy metal link to Diabetes

According to one study, Mercury exposure may increase the risk of developing Diabetes Type 2. Mercury appears to damage the pancreatic cells responsible for insulin production (Beta Cells) – meaning it could also play a role in Type 1. Mercury exposure can come from fish such as tuna, swordfish and shark meat as well as mercury dental fillings.

Studies have suggested that Arsenic, Cadmium, and Nickel also play a role in damaging Beta cells, reducing insulin levels and increasing blood glucose levels.

Solution

My advice is to eat organic, avoid junk food and consume foods and herbs that assist in removing heavy metals from the body. Emerging research shows that herbs such as Cilantro and Chlorella are able to bind to and excrete heavy metals from the body.

Consider adding Cilantro and Chlorella to your diet or supplementing.

Ayurvedic Perspective on Diabetes Mellitus

Ayurveda is the oldest medical science in existence, dating back several thousand years. Ayurvedic medicinal herbs, compounds, and treatment protocols have been tested in literally thousands of studies including clinical trials and case studies and have demonstrated significantly beneficial effects in hundreds of health conditions.

Descriptions of Diabetes Mellitus in Ayurvedic texts go back several thousand years in the books known as "Sushruta Samhita" and "Charaka Samhita". Diabetes Mellitus is referred to as "Madhu-Meha" - which is considered a urinary disorder due to the presence of sugar in the urine. Therefore, it is classified under a group of disorders referred to as "Prameha" which translates to "Urinary disorders".

In this chapter, I will be discussing the pathogenesis of "Prameha" in its relation to the development of Diabetes Mellitus.

Etiology

The main causes according to Ayurveda are basically a lack of exercise and poor dietary habits involving the excess consumption of foods that increase fat tissue, urinary output, and muscle energy – such as curd, sweet foods, and other high carbohydrate meals.

Classification of Diabetes Type 2 Based on Presentation:

1. Lean Diabetics
2. Obese Diabetics

The reason for this classification is the difference in pathogenesis.

It is also classified based on causes:

1. Congenital
2. Dietary/Lifestyle Related

Understanding Pathogenesis in Ayurveda

In order to understand the pathogenesis from an Ayurvedic perspective, you must first understand at least some part of the Ayurvedic understanding of physiology - this starts with **Doshas**.

Doshas are basically groups of physiological systems and activities that tend to work together. Doshas include various system's functions along with their secretions, enzymes and other biochemical constituents responsible for regulating their functions.

When certain aspects of these Doshas increase, decrease, or function abnormally, it results in the development of disease.

Please note that the concept of Doshas alone would take an entire book to describe and explain, however, I have tried to consolidate and explain them simply in a few brief paragraphs. Keep in mind that this is barely the tip of the iceberg when it comes to this topic.

Doshas are classified into 3 major categories:

1. Vata

This refers primarily to the nervous system and its functions such as the induction and regulation of processes such as circulation, respiration, peristalsis, excretion, orgasm, and literally every movement in the body. Therefore, it is connected to each of these systems. All types of signaling in the body are carried out via its function. It regulates every movement right down to blinking, moving, heartbeat, etc.

2. Pitta

This refers primarily to the metabolic functions responsible for breaking down nutrients - digestion, catabolic actions, and the means via which enzymates are released (through gastric secretions, etc) as well as certain metabolic hormones (Insulin, Ghrelin, Leptin, Glucagon, etc). It is also responsible for thermal control and all methods of processing – mental (neurotransmitters), visual (Photoreception), digestive (metabolic & Thyroid function), etc.

3. Kapha

This refers to the metabolic functions responsible for energy production at a tissue level (Glycogen), growth factors/hormones (GH, Testosterone, Estrogen, Progesterone, IGF, etc). It is also responsible for protection via lubrication with liquid substances (Synovial fluid for joints, cerebrospinal fluid for the brain, surfactant fluid for lungs, and mucin for the stomach), etc.

Ayurvedic Pathogenesis of Prameha, with relation to the developement of Diabetes Mellitus

It starts with all three doshas becoming dysregulated :

- Vata problems related to insulin signaling
- Pitta problems related to metabolic hormones
- Kapha problems related to energy production

In the beginning, Kapha tends to play a centralized role related to an increase in what is known as "Kleda" or moisture. It is a known thing that when glucose fills up cells in the form of glycogen, it does so together with a large amount of water. When glucose is not being absorbed, energy (glycogen) is not stored and the glucose passes through the kidneys as they filter the blood.

The excess glucose is then excreted via the urine and draws more fluids along with it. This is how the symptom of "Polyuria" develops as well as the symptoms of polydipsia and weakness. This is one of the reasons that Ayurveda consideres this condition to be related to the urinary system.

Back when this Ayurvedic theory of Diabetes originated, the diagnosis would be made based on sugar content in the urine as well as polyuria, therefore it was considered to be a disease affecting the urinary tract and kidneys.

<u>At the time of full manifestion of the disease, Vata becomes more predominant</u> as symptoms associated with Vata dosha arise - such as neuropathy, retinopathy, nephropathy, nutrient deficiencies, poor circulation, etc. In the classification of Prameha, Diabetes Mellitus (Madhu-Meha) is classified as a Vata predominant form of disease.

Pitta dysregulation plays a role throughout the pathogenesis in a more subtle way as it is what regulates the metabolic functions – due to being unable to carry out its function, sugar is not coverted to glycogen. When this condition is developing, the dysregulation of these 3 doshas affect multiple organs and tissues, namely:

- Meda, which means Fat (Increases due to more circulating insulin)
- Mamsa, which means Muscle (Starves due to inability to absorb glucose, potassium or amino acids)
- Majja, which means brain and nerves (Degeneration and neuropathy)
- Rakta, which means blood (Increased sugar causing Hyperglycemia)
- Lasika, which means lymph (Weakened immune system)

In Ayurveda, it is stated that majority of the changes take place during fat tissue metabolism (medovaha srotas) and in urine formation (mutravaha srotas).

Ayurveda also suggests that as Diabetes progresses, it causes a reduction in Ojas (compares to Adenosine Triphosphate) – it is a known thing in physiology that glucose molecules get converted into Adenosine Triphosphate for cellular energy. The lack of ATP results in debility and degeneration.

Symptoms of "Prameha" including Diabetes:

- Change in Quantitiy and Color of Urine
- Turbid Urine
- Excess Thirst
- Burning of Hands and Feet
- Heaviness
- Lethargy
- Sugar Presence in Urine
- Stickiness of Body

Treatment

I have mentioned several of the treatment options utilized in Ayurveda in the chapter on Herbal Medicines. One of the most praised medicines in classical Ayurveda is "Shilajit" or Mineral Pitch. The physician known as Sushruta (2600 BC) made the bold statement that Shilajit can cure many illness including Madhu-Meha (Diabetes Mellitus).

As you will see in the section on Shilajit, there is clinical evidence supporting its use in treating Diabetes.

Evidence-Based Herbal Medicines

All herbs, foods, and Ayurvedic formulations mentioned in this book have been used successfully in <u>clinical studies</u> as well as my clinical experience.

Sage

Sage (Salvia Officinalis), a common culinary herb, has a history of medicinal uses dating back to the ancient Greek and Egyptian civilizations. Sage has recently gotten much appreciation for its use in Alzheimer's disease, which as discussed earlier, is actually being classified as Diabetes Type 3 based on the role sugar metabolism plays in the pathogenesis of the disease. Sage has also demonstrated significant blood sugar lowering effects in Diabetes Type 2.

Based on pharmacological evidence, Sage appears to possess the following properties:

- Anti-oxidant
- Anti-cancer
- Anti-inflammatory
- Anti-nociceptive
- Anti-microbial
- Anti-mutagenic
- Anti-dementia
- Hypoglycemic
- Hypolipidemic

Its uses in folk medicine include:

- Ulcers
- Diarrhea
- Dizziness
- Tremors
- Gout
- Rheumatism
- Inflammation
- Hyperglycemia
- Paralysis
- Throat Infections
- Dental Abscesses
- Spasmodic Pain

Clinical evidence supports its use in:

- Diabetes Type 2
- Alzheimer's Disease
- Menopause
- High Cholesterol
- Pharyngitis
- Pain
* It has also been used for Memory Enhancement

Use in Diabetes

In clinical trials (Including Randomized placebo-controlled clinical trials) patients with Diabetes Type 2 being treated with Sage experienced significant improvement in several aspects of both blood sugar as well as blood lipids.

Clinical trials had the following results:

Reduction of:

- Fasting Blood Glucose
- Postprandial Blood Sugar
- HbA1c
- Total Cholesterol
- LDL-C

Increase of:

- HDL-C

Based on these results, its can be said that Sage holds much potential in managing blood sugar levels in Diabetes Type 2.

Dosage

According to studies:

1. 150mg Sage Leaf Extract, thrice daily for three months

2. 500mg Sage Leaf Extract, every eight hours for three months

In my experience:

500mg Sage Leaf Extract, twice or thrice daily has been effective

Side-effects

In clinical research on patients with Diabetes Type 2 taking Sage, no adverse effects were reported.

- Excessive or prolonged use of ethanolic extract and volatile oil may potential result in unwanted side-effects including vomiting, increased heart rate, allergic reactions, vertigo, hot flushes and several other unwanted symptoms.

- Therefore, one should use this with caution and by following the dosage recommended by their holistic physician.

Mode of Action

- Based on experimental research, Sage appears to work by inhibiting gluconeogenesis and increasing the action of insulin.

Amla

Amla is commonly known as Gooseberry or Indian Gooseberry. It is also sometimes referred to as "Amalaki" or its botanical name "Emblica Officinalis". Amla is a fruit known for its rich Vitamin C content and is often consumed in India for improving immunity and for anti-aging.

I personally recommend people to use supplements rather than consume the fruit as it is extremely sour in taste and many patients are unable to manage it even when used as a powder. My recommendation is a supplement that is not an extract, but rather a whole fruit supplement.

Based on pharmacological studies, Amla appears to possess the following properties:

- Hypoglycemic
- Hypolipidemic
- Anti-bacterial
- Anti-microbial
- Anti-oxidant
- Anti-inflammatory
- Anti-pyretic
- Analgesic
- Adaptogenic
- Hepatoprotective
- Anti-tumor
- Anti-ulcerogenic
- Gastroprotective

Its uses in Ayurvedic medicine include:

- Anemia
- Diabetes
- Gout
- Hepatitis
- Jaundice
- Premature Aging
- Hair Loss

- Fever
- Constipation
- Hemorrhaging
- Bronchitis
- Heart Disease
- Vision Problems
- General Debility
- Anti-aging
- Poor Appetite
- Acidity

Clinical evidence supports its use in:

- Diabetes Type 2
- High Cholesterol
- NERD (Non-Erosive Reflux Disease)
- Acidity*
- Anemia
- High Triglycerides
- Diabetic Retinopathy*

* In these cases, Amla is combined with other herbs or used in formulations where Amla is the key ingredient (E.g. Triphala).

Use in Diabetes

In clinical trials (Including Randomized placebo-controlled clinical trials) patients with Diabetes Type 2 being treated with Amla experienced significant improvement in several aspects of blood sugar, blood lipids, and Oxidative stress.

Clinical trials had the following results:

Reduction of:

- Fasting Blood Glucose
- Postprandial Blood Sugar
- HbA1c
- Total Cholesterol
- LDL-C

- Triglycerides
- C-reactive Protein

Increase of:

- HDL-C

Amla also demonstrated improvement in bio-markers of oxidative stress.

Based on these results, its can be said that Amla holds much potential in reducing blood sugar levels in Diabetes Type 2.

Dose

According to studies:

1. 1-3grams whole Amla, daily for three months

2. 250mg-500mg of Amla aqueous extract, twice daily

In my experience:

1000mg, thrice daily, before meals appears to work well. However, the dose has to be determined subjectively. Some patients may experience loose stools – dose must be lowered.

Side-effects

- In clinical research on patients with Diabetes Type 2 taking Amla, no adverse effects were reported.

- In my experience, Amla can sometimes cause strong hunger within minutes of consumption so I advise eating soon after taking it.

- In some cases, Amla can cause temporary, mild nausea shortly after consumption.

- In higher doses, Amla can cause diarrhea as it is a mild laxative. Determining the dose for amla is subjective, and in most cases, Amla is not used alone – Therefore it should be used under the supervision of an Ayurvedic doctor.

Mode of Action

Based on experimental research, Amla appears to work via regeneration and rejuvenation of the Beta Cells in the pancreas – leading to an increase in insulin production as well as secretion. Amla also contains Chromium, which appears to improve insulin sensitivity. In addition to its anti-diabetic effects, Amla also appears to inhibit Aldose Reductase – an enzyme that seems to play a key role in the development of diabetic complications.

Gymnema Sylvestre

Gymnema Sylvestre, also known as "Gurmar", is an Ayurvedic herb used for treating both Diabetes Type 1 and Type 2. In recent times, Gymnema has been named "The sugar destroyer" due to the fact that it not only reduces blood sugar but also temporarily blocks the ability to taste anything sweet.

This herb contains a chemical known as Gymnemic acid – which has shown potential to stimulate beta cells to release insulin as well as potential to assist in regeneration with long-term use. For this reason, Gymnema is considered a boon for insulin-dependent diabetics.

Based on pharmacological evidence, Gymnema Sylvestre appears to possess the following properties:

- Hypoglycemic
- Anti-arthritic
- Anti-bacterial
- Anti-microbial
- Anti-biotic
- Anti-inflammatory
- Anti-Cancer & Cytotoxic
- Anti-Hyperlipidemic
- Hepatoprotective
- Immunostimulant
- Wound Healing Agent

Its uses in Ayurvedic Medicine include:

- Diabetes
- Obesity
- Hepatomegaly
- Splenomegaly
- Kidney Stones
- Amenorrhea
- General Debility
- Typhoid Fever
- Common Cold

Clinical evidence supports its use in:

- Diabetes Type 1
- Diabetes Type 2
- Obesity

Use in Diabetes

In clinical studies, patients with Diabetes Type 2 & Type 1 being treated with Gymnema Sylvestre experienced significant improvement in several aspects of blood sugar metabolism.

Clinical studies demonstrated the following results:

Type 2 Diabetics experienced a reduction in:

- Fasting Blood Glucose
- Postprandial Blood Glucose
- HbA1c
- Fatigue
- Polyphagia

Type 1 Diabetics experienced a reduction in:

- Fasting Blood Glucose
- Postprandial Blood Glucose
- HbA1c
- There was also a reduction in insulin requirements

Dose

According to studies

400mg-500mg of the herb extract daily, for 3 months

In my experience:

Whole herb: 1-2 grams twice a day

Extract Supplement: 250mg, twice a day, with meals

Side-effects

In clinical research on patients with Diabetes Type 1 & 2 taking Gymnema Sylvestre, no adverse effects were reported.

- In my experience, Gymnema has sometimes caused mild heart burn – in such cases, I gave Amla together with Gymnema.

- In my research, I have come across one case of drug-induced liver injury. However, during my training and practice I have not come across a single patient whom experienced this side-effect, even with long-term use.

Mode of Action

Gymnema appears to work by stimulating the Beta cells in the pancreas to increase insulin production as well as secretion.

Cinnamon

Cinnamon is a common aromatic spice obtained from the bark of the Cinnamomum trees. The most common form found is stores is Cassia Cinnamon, which is often frowned upon due to its "Coumarin" content. Coumarin is a blood thinning component that can potentially damage the liver if used in large quantities.

Ceylon cinnamon is the more preferred form and it is sometimes called "True Cinnamon", however, it is just a safer option to the cassia variety.

In my opinion, both forms are beneficial for Diabetes.

Based on pharmacological evidence, Cinnamon appears to possess the following properties:

- Hypoglycemic
- Anti-inflammatory
- Anti-oxidant
- Anti-ulcer
- Anti-microbial
- Memory Booster
- Anti-coagulant
- Anti-bacterial
- Anti-fungal
- Anti-cancer
- Anti-mutagenic
- Anti-septic
- Anti-parasitic

Its uses in Ayurvedic & Folk Medicine include:

- Diabetes
- Gingivitis
- Diarrhea
- Congestion
- Bronchitis
- Pain
- Headache

- Vomiting
- Poor Appetite
- Rhinitis
- Dyspnea
- Piles

Clinical evidence supports is use in:

- Diabetes Type 2
- Menstrual Regulation in PCOS
- Reducing Total Cholesterol
- Reducing LDL-C
- Reducing Triglycerides

Use in Diabetes

In clinical trials (Including Randomized placebo-controlled clinical trials), patients with Diabetes Type 2 being treated with Cinnamon experienced significant improvement in several aspects of blood sugar and blood lipid levels.

Clinical trials had the following results:

Reduction of:

- Fasting Blood Glucose
- Postprandial Blood Sugar
- HbA1c
- Total Cholesterol, LDL-C & Triglycerides

Dose

According to studies

- Ceylon Cinnamon Extract – 1000mg before a meal
- Cassia Cinnamon – Up to 2 grams, thrice daily, for 20 days

In my experience

- Cassia Cinnamon – Up to 1 gram, thrice daily together with a hepatoprotective supplement such as LiverCare by Himalaya. I have used up to 5 grams of cinnamon daily for no more than 8 weeks.

- Ceylon – 500mg-750mg up to three times daily, before meals.

Side-effects

- In clinical research involving patients with Diabetes Type 2 taking Cinnamon, no adverse effects were reported.

- Can cause blood thinning, liver damage (Cassia), allergic reactions, skin irritation (if applied topically),

- In animal studies, coumarin (Cassia) increased the risk of cancer.

- Some people experience mouth sores from excess consumption

- May irritate the throat and cause coughing

- Can interact with other medicines such as blood thinners and other hepatotoxic drugs such as statins and acetaminophen (Paracetamol).

Mode Of Action

- Appears to inhibit Alpha-amylase – an enzyme responsible for absorbing carbohydrates.

- Cinnamon also increases GLUT4 receptors, insulin receptors and insulin receptor substrates – this improves the absorption of glucose in skeletal muscle and adipose tissue.

- Activates phosphorylation on the insulin receptor beta-subunit on fat cells via the activity of a proanthocyanidin in Cinnamon known as Cinnamtannin B1.

Vinegar

One of the common remedies that people come across for blood sugar and weight loss is Vinegar, more so Apple cider vinegar. Vinegar is basically a sour-tasting liquid that is made by fermentation. It contains about 5-20% acetic acid, and is linked to several health benefits.

The history of vinegar actually goes back thousands of years to the Egyptians and Babylonians. The medicinal value of vinegar has also been known for centuries for the treatment of wounds, poison ivy, croup, and digestive complaints.

Based on pharmacological evidence, Vinegar appears to possess the following properties:

- Anti-diabetic
- Anti-obesity
- Anti-bacterial
- Anti-cholesterol
- Anti-acidity
- Anti-hypertensive
- Anti-cancer

Its uses in Folk Medicine include:

- Diabetes Type 2
- High Cholesterol
- Acne and wounds
- Warts
- Allergies
- Weight Loss
- Heart Burn
- High Blood Pressure
- Coughs and Colds

Clinical Evidence supports its use in:

- Diabetes Type 2
- Varicose Veins

- Weight Loss
- Acne Scarring

Use in Diabetes

In clinical studies, patients with Diabetes Type 2 being treated with Vinegar or Apply cider vinegar experienced significant improvement in several aspects of blood sugar regulation.

Clinical trials had the following results:

Reduction of:

- Fasting Blood Glucose (Mild Reduction)
- Postprandial Blood Sugar
- Insulin

Side-effects

Several side-effects have been noted in cases studies. In multiple of these cases, it involved the consumption of <u>very large amounts</u> of apple cider vinegar daily. Side-effects included tooth erosion, low potassium, bone loss.

Other side-effects include reduced appetite and delayed gastric emptying – this may worsen conditions such as gastroperesis.

Skin burns and throat burns have also been noted.

Appears to delay gastric emptying – avoid in gastroparesis

Mode of Action

- Vinegar appears to improve insulin-stimulated glucose uptake in skeletal muscles by increasing the rate of glycogen synthesis.

Salacia Chinensis & Salacia Oblonga

Known as Saptarangi in Ayurvedic medicine, Salacia Chinensis and its relative Salacia Oblonga are well known for their medicinal benefits. Salacia Chinensis is sometimes referred to as Chinese Salacia as it grows predominantly in China (as well as Vietnam, Malaysia, Sri Lanka and other South East Asian countries). Salacia Oblonga, its relative, is commonly found in Sri Lanka and is known by the name "Saptachakra".

In recent times, Salacia Chinensis and Salacia Oblonga have become well known in Ayurvedic medicine as some of the most effective herbs for fighting Diabetes and Obesity. They contains Salicinol and Kotalanol – two potent Alpha-Glucosidase inhibitors - inhibiting these prevents the absorption of carbohydrates in the intestine.

Taking this herb before meals is the best way to prevent carbohydrate absorption, which also helps prevent weight gain.

Based on pharmacological evidence, Salacia herbs appear to possess the following properties:

- Anti-diabetic
- Anti-obesity
- Anti-cholesterol
- Alpha-Glucosidase Inhibitor
- Cardioprotective
- Hepatoprotective
- Nephroprotective

Its uses in Ayurvedic medicine include:

- Diabetes
- Pain & Swelling
- Piles
- Skin disorders
- Rhinitis

- Hives
- Amenorrhea
- Liver Disorders

Clinical evidence supports its use in:

- Diabetes Type 2
- Obesity

Use in Diabetes

In clinical studies, healthy patients as well as patients with Diabetes Type 2 being treated with Salacia Chinensis or Salacia Oblonga experienced significant improvement in several aspects of blood sugar regulation. It also had significant results in a study on weight loss.

Clinical trials had the following results:

Reduction of:

- Postprandial Blood Sugar
- Postprandial Insulin
- HbA1c (Slight Reduction)

Dose:

According to studies:

200mg-1000mg – the higher dose was used frequently for blocking glucose absorption . This supplement tends to be used for simply preventing glucose spikes after meals in most studies.

In my experience:

500mg-1000mg of 20:1 extract, up to 2 times daily before meals.

NOTE: In my opinion, this herb has the potential to control blood sugar levels by blocking carbohydrate absorption, but I do not think of it as a treatment option due to the lack of evidence in long-term use. It is however, a good way to help diabetics enjoy some of their favorite meals without blood sugar spikes – of course, depending on the quantity of carbohydrates, it may need to be used in combination with other anti-diabetic herbs.

Side-effects

In clinical research with patients taking Salacia Oblonga or Salacia Chinensis, no severe adverse effects were reported.

However, mild side-effects such as flatulence, abdominal pain and nausea have been noted.

In my clinical experience, an increase in gas has been a fairly common side-effect.

Mode of Action

Inhibits an enzyme known as Alpha-Glucosidase, thus slowing down the absorption of carbohydrates. This helps to prevent blood sugar spikes and also assists in weight loss.

European Ash (Fraxinus Excelsior)

Known a Common Ash or European Ash, this herb has been used for several health conditions over the centuries. Throughout Europe there have been historical references describing the uses of European Ash for medicinal purposes. Even the great Greek physician Hippocrates mentioned the medicinal use of it.

Based on pharmacological evidence, herbology references, historical references and other medicinal plant databases, European Ash appears to possess the following properties:

- Anti-rheumatic
- Anti-hypertensive
- Anti-pyretic
- Anti-diabetic
- Anti-microbial
- Anti-inflammatory
- Neuroprotective
- Anti-diarrheal

Uses in traditional medicine:

- Gout
- Fevers
- Diarrhea
- Uterine Fibroids
- Burns
- Scalds
- Anuria
- Rheumatoid Arthritis

Clinical evidence supports its use in:

- Diabetes Type 2

Use in Diabetes

In clinical studies (including a randomized, double-blind, placebo-controlled crossover study), patients with common risk-factors for Diabetes that were treated with Fraxinus Excelsior experienced significant improvement in multiple aspects of blood sugar regulation. A decrease in fat mass was also seen.

Clinical trials had the following results:

Reduction of:

- Postprandial Blood Sugar
- Fat Mass

Increase of:

- Postprandial Insulin secretion
- Adiponectin:leptin ratio

Dose

According to studies:

333mg of Flaxinus Excelsior Seed Extract, thrice daily, for three weeks

In my experience:

1000mg of Flaxinus Excelsior Seed Extract (Glucevia), twice daily, after meals. In some cases, up to three times daily after food.

Side-effects

In clinical research no adverse effects were reported. Some references suggest the possibility of allergic reactions when consumed in excess.

Berberine

Berberine is a potent anti-diabetic compound that is found in plants such as Barberry, Tinospora Cordifolia, Goldenseal, Oregon Grape and Chinese Goldthread. Most of these sources are predominantly used for the purposes of fighting off infections as well as digestive complaints.

Berberine is getting quite a bit of attention in the natural health community, as a supplement that provides benefits similar to, if not, more effective than pharmaceutical drugs used for treating Diabetes.

Berberine is literally my first choice for managing Diabetes Type 2 due to the significant blood glucose improvements I've seen in clinical use.

Based on pharmacological evidence, Berberine (and its herbal sources) appear to possess the following properties:

- Anti-diabetic
- Anti-hypertensive
- Hepatoprotective
- Anti-cancer
- Anti-hyperlipidemic
- Anti-microbial
- Anti-inflammatory
- Anti-depressive
- Anti-oxidant
- Anti-obesity

Uses of Berberine's herbal sources in Ayurvedic and Chinese medicine include:

- Diabetes
- Fatty Liver Disease
- Obesity
- Infections
- Heart Disease
- Eye Disease

- Chyluria
- Skin Diseases
- Dysuria
- Oral infections
- Ulcers

Clinical evidence supports its use in:

- Diabetes Type 2
- High Cholesterol
- Obesity
- SIBO
- Cardiac Health
- Canker Sores
- Fatty Liver Disease

Use in Diabetes

In clinical studies (including a randomized, double-blind placebo-controlled clinical trial), patients with Diabetes Type 2 and Metabolic syndrome being treated with Berberine experienced significant improvement in several aspects of blood sugar regulation as well as blood lipids.

It has also been useful in weight reduction.

Clinical trials had the following results:

Reduction of:

- Fasting Blood Sugar
- Postprandial Blood Sugar
- Fasting Insulin
- HbA1c
- Total Cholesterol
- LDL-C
- Triglycerides
- Waist Circumference

Increase of:

- HDL (Slight Raise)
- Insulin Sensitivity (in patients with NAFLD)

Dose:

According to studies:

On average, 1500mg daily, in divided doses before meals for up to 24 weeks.

In my experience:

Same as studies - 500mg, thrice daily, before food.

Side-effects

Generally safe, however, high doses may potentially cause gastrointestinal side-effects such as abdominal discomfort, mild diarrhea or even constipation – all of which appear to be dose-dependent.

In my experience, Berberine may cause hypoglycemia if combined with other anti-diabetic herbs, supplements or medicines.

Drug interactions are potential with macrolide antibiotics such as Azithromycin as well as statins.

I also advise avoiding its use during pregnancy.

Mode of Action

Appears to activate the enzyme known as Adenosine Monophosphate-activated Protein Kinase (AMPK) and inhibit Protein-Tyrosine Phosphatase 1B (PTP1B). Increases the activity of low-activity glucose transporter GLUT1. It also appears to inhibit the enzyme aldose reductase, suggesting it may prevent or treat diabetic complications.

Nigella Sativa

Also known as black seed, Nigella Sativa has become a very popular supplement for a wide-range of conditions including weight loss, thyroid conditions and liver disorders. It has a long history of medicinal uses in India, Persia, Greece and Egypt. In recent times, it has been utilized in hundreds of studies and is quickly gaining attention for its vast range of medicinal benefits.

It is also referred to as Black Cumin, Kalonji, and Black Caraway.

According to studies, it possesses the following pharmacological properties:

- Anti-diabetic
- Anti-cancer
- Immunomodulator
- Analgesic
- Anti-microbial
- Anti-inflammatory
- Spasmolytic
- Bronchodilator
- Hepatoprotective
- Renal Protective
- Gastro-Protective
- Anti-oxidant
- Anti-obesity
- Diuretic

Its uses in Ayurvedic medicine and other medical sciences include:

- Diabetes Type 2
- Hypothyroidism
- Diarrhea
- Hepatitis
- Alopecia
- Jaundice
- Headache
- Round Worms
- Aphrodisiac

- Asthma
- Bronchitis
- Amenorrhea
- Dysmenorrhea
- Vomiting
- Rheumatism

Clinical evidence supports its use in:

- Diabetes Type 2
- High Cholesterol
- Hashimoto's Thyroiditis
- Hepatitis C
- Allergies

Use in Diabetes

In clinical studies (including a randomized, double-blind placebo-controlled clinical trial), patients with Diabetes Type 2 and Metabolic syndrome being treated with Nigella Sativa experienced significant improvement in several aspects of blood sugar regulation as well as blood lipids. It has also been useful in weight reduction in other studies.

Clinical trials had the following results:

Reduction of:

- Fasting Blood Sugar
- Fasting Insulin
- HbA1c
- Total Cholesterol
- LDL-C
- Triglycerides
- Blood Pressure

Increase of:

- HDL-C

Dose

<u>According to studies:</u>

- 2-3 grams of seeds or powder, daily for 12 weeks.

- 2.5ml of oil, twice daily, for 6 weeks.

<u>In my experience:</u>

- 3-5 grams of seeds daily, in divided doses, on an empty stomach

- 2.5ml of oil, twice daily, 30 minutes before food.

Side-effects

No major side-effects have been reported, however in my experience, large amounts can cause gastric discomfort, upset stomach and vomiting.

- Black seed may potentially slow blood clotting.

- If combined with other Diabetes medications, it may result in hypoglycemia.

Mode of Action

According to experimental research, Nigella Sativa appears to enhance insulin secretion by inducing beta cell proliferation and regeneration. Research also suggests that Nigella Sativa decreases gluconeogenesis in the liver, increases muscle GLUT4, and activates the AMPK pathway.

Stinging Nettle

This flowering plant has become a very popular herbal remedy with its medicinal benefits being validated in multiple clinical studies. In recent times, Stinging Nettle has become well known for managing allergies, prostate enlargement, hormone regulation and acne, but studies have also demonstrated its potential as a highly effective remedy for controlling blood sugar levels.

According to studies, it possesses the following pharmacological properties:

- Anti-histamine
- Anti-proliferative
- Hypoglycemic
- Anti-oxidant
- Hypolipidemic
- Anti-rheumatic
- Anti-cancer
- Anti-vital

Its been used in traditional, folk and herbal medicine for:

- Hair Loss
- Diabetes
- Gingivitis
- Diarrhea
- Allergies
- Wound Healing
- Hemorrhoids
- Insect Bites
- Anemia
- Kidney Disorders
- Asthma
- Congestion

Clinical evidence supports its use in:

- Diabetes Type 2
- Benign Prostate Enlargement
- Allergic Rhinitis

Use in Diabetes

In clinical studies, healthy patients as well as patients with Diabetes Type 2 being treated with Stinging Nettle experienced significant improvement in several aspects of blood sugar regulation as well as blood pressure and blood lipids.

Clinical trials had the following results:

Reduction of:

- Fasting Blood Sugar
- Postprandial Blood Sugar
- HbA1c
- Systolic Blood Pressure
- Triglycerides

Increase of:

- HDL-C

Dose

According to studies:

- 500mg of Nettle Leaf Extract, every 8 hours, for 3 months

- 10g daily of whole herb, divided into 3 doses, taken 15 minutes before food.

<u>In my experience:</u>

- 500mg of Nettle Leaf Extract, thrice daily, before meals.

Side-effects

Generally considered safe for use, however it may sometimes cause mild stomach upset, diarrhea, skin rash (when applied topically), fluid retention and sweating.

Drug interactions

- May interact with blood thinners, antihypertensives, diuretics, NSAIDS, Sedatives and Lithium

Mode of Action

In experimental studies, Stinging Nettle appears to inhibit the enzyme "alpha-glucosidase" and "alpha-amylase", thus slowing down carbohydrate absorption. It also appears to regenerate beta cells in the pancreas and prevent islet atrophy, thus improving plasma insulin levels.

Aloe Vera

In Ayurveda, Aloe Vera is called "Kumari", which roughly translates to "a young girl" - referring to its anti-aging properties. Aloe vera was used by the Greeks and ancient Egyptians whom also considered it to be the "Plant of Immortality" for the same reason.

The number of medicinal benefits associated with Aloe Vera are innumerable, as well as its multiple cosmetic uses. In recent studies, Aloe Vera has shown much promise for treating Diabetes.

According to studies, Aloe Vera possesses the following pharmacological properties:

- Anti-diabetic
- Anti-fungal
- Anti-inflammatory
- Wound Healing
- Anti-cancer
- Immunomodulator
- Anti-hyperlipidemic
- Anti-viral
- Anti-microbial

Aloe Vera has been used in Ayurvedic medicine and other traditional medicine systems for:

- Burns
- Wounds
- Headaches
- Psoriasis
- Intestinal Worms
- Jaundice
- Bronchitis
- Ascites
- Anemia
- Menstrual Irregularities
- Abscesses
- Asthma

- Nose Bleeds
- Poor Appetite
- Constipation
- Colic

Clinical evidence supports its use in:

- Diabetes Type 2
- Psoriasis
- Canker Sores
- Constipation
- Irritable Bowel Syndrome

Use in Diabetes

In clinical studies (including randomized, double-blind, placebo-controlled clinical trials), healthy patients as well as patients with Prediabetes and Early non-treated Diabetes Type 2 being treated with Aloe Vera experienced significant improvement in several aspects of blood sugar regulation.

Clinical trials had the following results:

Reduction of:

- Fasting Blood Sugar
- HbA1c
- Total Cholesterol & LDL-C
- Triglycerides

Increase of:

- HDL-C

Dose

According to studies

- 1 tablespoon of Aloe Vera juice, twice a day for 2 weeks

- 100mg-200mg Aloe Vera gel powder in divided doses. Eg. 50mg-100mg upon waking and 50mg-100mg before bed for 6 months

In my experience:

- Same as studies, however I have used doses up to 300mg twice a day in cases of extremely high blood glucose.

Side-effects

The most common side-effects are abdominal pain, cramping and muscle weakness. To avoid the abdominal pain and cramping, it is best to administer with ginger or ginger tea.

Mode of Action

Based on experimental studies, Aloe Vera appears to reduce hepatic gluconeogenesis. It also appears to stimulate the production and/or release of insulin from beta-cells.

Fig Leaves (Ficus Carica)

Figs are a popular fruit known for their ability to boost energy levels and regulate bowel movements. They are rich in nutrients such as calcium, manganese, magnesium, copper, iron, phosphorus, zinc, B-vitamins, and vitamin K, as well as antioxidant polyphenols which play an important role in combating oxidative stress.

Nowadays, Figs are popular as a dried fruit, jam, and cookie filling, however, the more imporant part of the fig tree for the purpose of blood sugar management, is the leaves.

Based on studies, Figs (and their phytonutrients) have the following pharmacological properties:

- Anti-oxidant
- Anti-diabetic
- Anti-cancer
- Anti-fungal
- Anti-bacterial
- Laxative
- Anti-spasmodic
- Cytotoxic
- Anti-inflammatory
- Hypolipidemic
- Anti-septic

Fig Tree's uses in Ayurvedic medicine and other traditional medical systems include:

- Diabetes
- Constipation
- Weakness
- High Blood Pressure

- Piles
- High cholesterol
- Low Libido
- Calluses
- Warts
- Parasites

Clinical evidence supports its use in:

- Diabetes Type 2 (Leaves)
- Constipation (Fruit)
- Atopic Dermatitis (Extract of fruit)
- Common Warts (Latex)

Use in Diabetes

In a double-blind, crossover clinical trial, patients with Diabetes Type 2 being treated with a Fig Leaf decoction experienced significant improvement in postprandial blood sugar.

The study suggests that a decoction of Fig Leaves may play an important role in reducing postprandial blood sugar when combined with oral hypoglycemic agents.

Dose

In the study:

Leaf extract prepared with 13 grams of dried leave powder, boiled in 500ml of water for 15 minutes, then cooled and filtered.

In my experience:

2 tablespoons, boiled in 1 cup of water until quantity of water reduces to 1/2. Then consumed in a dose of 100ml-150ml.

Side-effects

Generally considered safe, but may cause diarrhea in excessive use (of fruit).

- There is not enough evidence to suggest possible drug interactions or adverse effects at this time. However, in my research, I have found no evidence of any severe adverse effects.

Mode of Action

Research suggests that the blood sugar lowering effects of Ficus Carica may be due to the improvement of one or more of the following:
- Insulin receptors
- Insulin receptor substrates
- Glucose Transporters, etc.

Based on the the fact that Ficus Carica increased plasma insulin levels (in experimental studies), it is suggested that this herb may potentiate pancreatic insulin secretion.

In vitro studies have demonstrated inhibitory effects on the alpha-amylase and alpha-glucosidase enzymes, thus slowing down the absorption of carbohydrates.

Flax Seed

Flax seed is one the most well known remedies for digestive complaints such as constipation. It is rich in anti-oxidants, manganese, thiamine, magnesium, phosphorus, copper and selenium. It is also a great source of fiber and omega-3 fatty acids with a wide range of traditional as well as clinically evident health benefits, making it a functional food – meaning it has the potential to both nourish you as well as treat illneses.

Based on studies, Flax seeds have the following pharmacological properties:

- Anti-oxidant
- Anti-cancer
- Anti-diabetic
- Anti-viral
- Anti-bacterial
- Anti-inflammatory
- Anti-artherosclerotic
- Cardioprotective

Its use in traditional medical systems include:

- Constipation
- Boils & Abscesses
- Diarrhea
- Low Stamina
- Anti-aging
- Wound Healing
- Diuretic
- Cancer
- Bronchitis
- Nail disorder
- Freckles

- Abdominal Pain
- Asthma & Tuberculosis
- Haemoptysis
- Splenomegaly
- Ulcers
- Poor Memory
- Gingival Disorders

Clinical evidence supports its use in:

- Diabetes Type 2
- High Cholesterol
- Cancer
- Weight Loss
- Menopause
- High Blood Pressure

Use in Diabetes

In clinical studies (including an open-label clinical trial), healthy patients as well as patients with Diabetes Type 2 being treated with Flax Seeds experienced significant improvement in several aspects of blood sugar regulation as well as blood lipids. In these studies, flax seed powder was either supplemented or added to foods.

Clinical trials had the following results:

Reduction of:

- Fasting Blood Sugar
- HbA1c
- Total Cholesterol
- Triglycerides
- LDL-C

Increase of:

- HDL-C

Dose

<u>According to studies:</u>

- 10 grams of flax seed powder daily for 1 month

- 5 grams of flax seed gum daily, added to food for 3 months

<u>In my experience:</u>

- 1 tablespoon of flax seeds or powder, daily, as part of regular diet. (I recommend introducing flax seeds into your diet gradually)

Side-effects

In the beginning, due to the high fiber content, flax seeds may cause some gastric discomfort. To avoid this, I recommend starting with small amounts and increasing it daily. Together with this, drink ginger or fennel tea to help relieve these effects. May interact with NSAIDS, cholesterol lowering drugs and blood thinners. It may also inhibit the absorption of certain medications.

Mode of Action

Appears to improve glucose utilization in the liver and muscle tissues. Evidence indicates that it has a regenerative effect on the pancreatic islets that produce insulin and also plays a role in inhibiting the enzyme alpha-glucosidase.

Fenugreek

Fenugreek is one of the more interesting medicinal herbs I have come across due to its ability to improve multiple health complaints that are associated with aging such as high cholesterol, high blood sugar, constipation, low libido, menopause, low energy and digestive complaints.

Fenugreek has a long history of medicinal use for breast milk production, swollen joints, obesity, chronic fevers, and boils.

Fenugreek's nutritional profile includes iron, manganese, copper, magnesium, phosphorus and vitamin B6.

Based on studies, Fenugreek has the following pharmacological properties:

- Anti-diabetic
- Anti-bacterial
- Anti-fungal
- Anti-inflammatory
- Anti-oxidant
- Anti-cancer
- Anti-ulcer
- Anti-lithigenic
- Hypocholesterolemic
- Anti-lipidemic
- Hepatoprotective
- Galactogogue
- Anti-DHT
- Aphrodisiac

Its uses in Ayurveda and Traditional medicine include:

- Diabetes Type 2

- High Cholesterol
- Edema
- Low Libido
- Scanty Breast Milk
- Obesity
- Pyrexia
- Boils
- Bronchitis
- Dyspepsia & Weak Digestion
- Arthritis
- Sciatica
- Allergies

Clinical evidence supports its use in:

- Diabetes Type 1 & 2
- High Cholesterol
- Low Libido
- Low Milk Supply
- Benign Prostate Hyperplasia
- Hypertriglyceridemia
- Vaginal Dryness

Use in Diabetes

In clinical studies (including randomized, double-blind, placebo-controlled clinical trials), patients with Diabetes Type 1 & Type 2 being treated with Fenugreek experienced significant improvement in several aspects of blood sugar regulation as well as blood lipids.

Changes were also seen in urinary glucose levels

Clinical trials had the following results:

Reduction of:

- Fasting Blood Sugar
- Postprandial Blood Sugar
- Urinary Glucose
- HbA1c
- Total Cholesterol
- Triglycerides
- LDL-C

Increase of

- HDL-C

Dose

According to studies:

- 10 to 25 grams of seeds (or powdered seeds) daily mixed with food or yogurt for up to 8 weeks

- In one study, 100grams of defatted seed powder was used daily for 10 days.

- 1 gram of hydroalcoholic extract daily for 2 months

In my experience:

- Up to 25 grams of seeds daily, in divided doses, mixed with food

- 500mg Fenugreek Extract, twice daily, before meals.

Side-effects

- Fenugreek may induce an abortion so should be avoided during pregnancy.

- Some people may be allergic to fenugreek.

- More research is needed to confirm side-effects, however, in my experience I have seen no major side effects when used correctly under the proper guidance of a holistic doctor.

Mode of Action

Appears to work by stimulating insulin production and/or release from the pancreatic beta-cells. There is also evidence suggesting that fenugreek increases the activity of gluconeogenic enzymes.

Caucasian Whortleberry

Also known by its botanical name, Vaccinium Arctostaphylos, this berry has the potential to significantly reduce the symptoms of Diabetes Type 2.

Native to the middle east, Caucasian Whortleberry is not yet a well studied or well known fruit, however, it has already been used in a few clinical studies and demonstrated quite impressive results.

Based of what is currently known about it, Caucasian Whortleberry (and it's chemical constituents) appears to have the following pharmacological properties:

- Anti-oxidant
- Anti-inflammatory
- Anti-diabetic
- Hypocholesterolemic
- Anti-microbial
- Anti-bacterial

Uses in traditional medicine:

- Diabetes
- Hypertension

At this time, not much is known about this herb

Clinical evidence supports its use in:

- Diabetes Type 2
- Hyerlipidemia

Use in Diabetes

In a randomized, double-blind, placebo-controlled clinical trial, patients with Diabetes Type 2 being treated with Caucasian Whortleberry experienced significant improvement in several aspects of blood sugar regulation.

It has also demonstrated benefits in clinical studies involving patients with Hyperlipidemia.

Clinical trials had the following results:

Reduction of:

- Fasting Blood Sugar
- Postprandial Blood Sugar
- HbA1c
- Total Cholesterol
- Triglycerides
- LDL-C

Dose

According to studies:

- 350mg of Caucasian Whortleberry Hydroalcoholic Extract, every 8 hours, for 2 months.

In my experience:

- Clinically, I have only used it in a few cases. I have used it personally and with a few patients as a handful, on an empty stomach.

Side-effects

Currently unknown.

- In the clinical study with Diabetic patients, no effect on liver or kidney function was seen, nor were any adverse effects reported.

- Based off of pharmacological effects, it may interact with anti-diabetic and anti-cholesterol medications.

Note

Caucasian Whortleberry is not to be confused with Bilberry as these are two different berries, although they are related via the same family of plants.

Mode of Action

Experimental studies suggest that Caucasian Whortleberry works via the activation of protein kinase activating AMP (AMPK) to reduce blood glucose levels.

Walnut Leaf

Known as "Akshotaka" in Ayurveda and botanically as Juglans Regia, the Walnut tree is held in high regard for its medicinal properties. Walnuts themselves are actually seeds that are contained within a fruit which is also used for medicinal purposes along with the leaves and bark.

Walnuts themselves are rich in various minerals, vitamins and polyunsaturated fatty acids. However, in the case of treating Diabetes, the leaves are needed for consumption.

Based on studies, the Walnut Tree leaves (and its chemical constituents) possess the following pharmacological properties:

- Anti-diabetic
- Anti-bacterial
- Analgesic
- Anti-Rheumatism
- Anti-fungal
- Anodyne
- Cytotoxic
- Anti-microbial

Uses of the Walnut Tree and its various parts in Ayurvedic and Traditional medicine systems include:

- Gum bleeding (Leaves)
- Dental Plaque (Leaves)
- Swelling (Fruit)
- Glandular Swelling (Fruit)
- Pain (Fruit)
- Insomnia (Oil)
- General Debility (Fruit)
- Emaciation (Fruit)

- Sexual Debility (Fruit and Walnut)
- Constipation (Walnut)
- Tape Worms (Oil)
- Dry Cough (Fruit)

Clinical evidence supports its use in:

- Diabetes Type 2
- High Blood Pressure
- Age-related Cognitive Impairment
- Cardiovascular Risk Factors
- Fertility (Males)

Use in Diabetes

In a randomized, double-blind, placebo-controlled clinical trial, patients with Diabetes Type 2 being treated with Walnut Leaf Extract experienced significant improvement in several aspects of blood sugar regulation as well as blood lipids

Clinical trials had the following results:

Reduction of:

- Fasting Blood Sugar
- Postprandial Blood Sugar
- HbA1c
- Total Cholesterol
- Triglycerides

Dose

According to the study:

- 100mg, twice daily for three months

In my experience:

- 1 teaspoon of dried leafs in one cup of boiling water and let steep for 15 minutes. This is taken 2-3 times daily.

Side-effects

Leaves have no known side effects.

- Might cause low blood sugar if used in large quantities.

- Not enough research is available to know the potential side-effects.

- Use with caution and with the medical supervision of a holistic physician.

Mode of Action

In experimental studies, Walnut leaf was able to increase the number of pancreatic beta-cells as well as insulin secretion. It also appears to inhibit hepatic gluconeogenesis.

Jackfruit Leaf

Known as "Panasa" in Ayurvedic medicine, and botanically as Artocarpus Heterophyllus, this plant can be considered as a functional food due to the fact that it is both highly nutritious as well as useful for treating various health conditions. Nowadays, the fruit has become quite popular as a meat substitute in the vegan and vegetarian communities.

In the case of Diabetes, the leaves are used.

Based on studies, the Jackfruit plant appears to have the following pharmacological properties:

- Anti-oxidant
- Hypolipidemic
- Anti-diabetic
- Anti-pyretic
- Analgesic
- Immunomodulator
- Anti-tumor

Its uses in Ayurveda and traditional medical systems include:

- Diarrhea
- Asthma
- Convulsions
- Wounds
- Inflammation
- Diabetes
- Pyrexia
- Weakness
- Bell's Palsy
- Low Sperm Count

Clinical evidence supports its use in:

- Diabetes Type 2
- Bell's Palsy

Use in Diabetes

In an interventional, single-blind clinical trial, patients with Diabetes Type 2 being treated with Jackfruit Leaf Aqueous Extract experienced significant improvement in several factors related to blood sugar metabolism and Diabetes symptoms.

Clinical trials had the following results:

Reduction of:

- Fasting Blood Sugar
- Postprandial Blood Sugar
- HbA1c
- Total Cholesterol
- Diabetes symptoms
    - Polyuria
    - Polydipsia
    - Polyphagia
    - Lassitude
    - Joint pain
    - Excessive sweating
    - Dryness of mouth

Dose

According to study:

- 96ml, four times a day, after food, for 30 days.

<u>In my experience:</u>

- 50-100ml, three to four times daily, after food.

Side-effects

No adverse effects were seen in the study, nor in my experience.

- May interact with diabetes medications or anti-cholesterol medications.

- May cause hypoglycemia in high doses or when combined with other anti-diabetic medications.

Mode of Action

Based on experimental studies, Jackfruit leaf extract appears to stimulate the release of insulin from remaining pancreatic Beta cells.

Withania Coagulans

Known as "Rishyagandha" in Ayurveda, this herb helps improve blood sugar levels quite effectively, especially when combined with Fenugreek. Withania Coagulans berries are quite popular in India for their ability to clot milk for cheese production and in North India for treating Diabetes.

In Ayurveda, Rishyagandha is considered a nourishing herb and is mentioned in the classical Ayurvedic text "Charaka Samhita" in the Sutra-Stana section, Chapter 4, verse 9.

Based on studies, Withania Coagulans appears to have the following pharmacological properties:

- Anti-diabetic
- Anti-stress
- Anti-oxidant
- Nephroprotective
- Hepatoprotective
- Hypolipidemic
- CNS Depressant
- Anti-tumor
- Anti-inflammatory
- Wound Healing
- Immuno-suppressive
- Anti-fungal
- Anti-bacterial

Uses in Ayurvedic medicine and traditional medical systems:

- Diabetes
- Emaciation
- Asthma
- Lumbago

- Opthalmia
- Piles
- Insomnia
- Colic
- Toothache

Clinical evidence supports its use in:

- Diabetes Mellitus Type 2

Use in Diabetes

In a clinical study, patients with Diabetes Type 2 being treated with Withania Coagulans fruit powder experienced significant improvement in blood sugar regulation and diabetes symptoms.

Clinical trials had the following results:

Reduction of:

- Fasting Blood Sugar
- Postprandial Blood Sugar
- Total Cholesterol
- Diabetes symptoms
    - Polyuria
    - Polydipsia
    - Polyphagia
    - Weakness
    - Joint pain
    - Burning
    - Tingling Sensation

Dose

According to studies:

- 10 grams of fruit powder daily, divided in 2 doses

- Combination of 10 seeds of Withania Coagulans and 6 grams of Fenugreek in 150ml of water, twice daily for 90 days.

In my experience:

- 10 grams of fruit powder daily, divided into 2 doses. I have found that it combines well with Fenugreek, Sage or Triphala.

Side-effects

No side-effects were seen in studies.

- Based on pharmacological evidence, it may interact with anti-diabetic, anti-cholesterol, and immuno-suppressive drugs.

Mode of Action

Appears to stimulate the glycolytic pathway and reduce gluconeogenesis. It also appears to enhance insulin secretion from beta cells.

Indian Gentian

Indian Gentian is quite a rare jewel, known as "Mammajak" in Ayurveda and "Enicostemma Littorale" botanically. It has been traditionally used for treating Diabetes, fevers, obesity and snake bites. It is commonly used in anti-diabetic formulations due to its potent blood sugar lowering properties.

In my experience, Indian Gentian works quite effectively as a single herb as well.

In studies, Indian Gentian appears to have the following pharmacological properties:

- Anti-diabetic
- Anti-bacterial
- Anti-inflammatory
- Anti-spasmodic
- Anti-hypertensive
- Anti-hyperlipidemic
- Hepatoprotective
- Anti-ulcer
- Anti-microbial
- Anti-oxidant

Its uses in Ayurvedic and Traditional medical systems include:

- Diabetes
- Fevers
- Low Appetite
- Snake Bites
- Obesity
- Skin Diseases
- Rheumatism

Clinical evidence supports its use in:

- Diabetes Type 2

Use in Diabetes

In an open randomized controlled clinical study, patients with Diabetes Type 2 being treated with Indian Gentian experienced significant improvement in blood sugar regulation and diabetes symptoms.

Clinical trials had the following results:

Reduction of:

- Fasting Blood Sugar
- Postprandial Blood Sugar
- Urinary Sugar
- HbA1c
- Total Cholesterol

Significant Improvement was seen in various symptoms of Diabetes:

- Excessive Sweating
- Burning of Feet
- Tingling Sensation
- Polyuria, Polydipsia, Polyphagia
- Weakness
- Joint Pain
- Loss of Libido

Another study demonstrated:

- Improved Kidney Function

- Improved Lipid Profile
- Improved Blood Pressure
- Prevention of progression of Diabetic complications

Dose

<u>According to studies:</u>

- 5 grams, twice daily, before breakfast and dinner with lukewarm water for 12 weeks.

- 500mg Mamajjaka Extract, twice daily, after meals, for 3 months.

<u>In my experience:</u>

- 2-3 grams, thrice daily, before meals with lukewarm water.

Side-effects

No side-effects were seen in studies.

- Based off of the pharmacological properties of this herb, it may interact with other diabetes medications

- It may results in hypoglycemia if used in excess.

Mode of Action

Appears to enhance glucose-induced insulin release from pancreatic islets via the K(+)-ATP channel dependent pathway. Also appears to reduce inflammatory responses associated with insulin resistance via the inhibition of pathways such as JNK & NF-kB. Also appears to restore expression of PPAR-y – thus enhancing insulin signalling.

American Ginseng

A very popular herb among Native Americans, this plants' root and leaves have been used for medicinally for various ailments. Research supports its use in Diabetes and memory enhancement. It used to grow abundantly in North America but is now predominantly grown in Ontario, throughout Canada and Wisconsin, USA.

In some American states, this herb is recognized as an endangered and/or threatened species

Based on studies, American Ginseng appears to possess the following pharmacological properties:

- Anti-diabetic
- Anti-osteoporosis
- Anti-obesity
- Anti-cancer
- Anti-hypertensive
- Anti-ischemic
- Anti-arrhymthmic
- Neuroprotective
- Neurotrophic
- Memory Boosting
- Adaptogenic

Its uses in Traditional medicine include:

- Weakness
- Asthenia
- Colitis
- Aging
- Cancer
- Senility

- Bleeding Disorders
- Atherosclerosis

Clinical evidence supports its use in:

- Diabetes Type 2
- Improving Memory
- Cold & Flu
- ADHD

Use in Diabetes

In multiple clinical studies, patients with Diabetes Type 2 as well as healthy individuals being treated with American Ginseng experienced significant improvement in blood sugar levels.

Clinical trials had the following results:

Reduction of:

- Postprandial Blood Sugar

*These effects appear to be time-dependent rather than dose dependent.

*The reduction in post-prandial blood sugar tends to be seen when American ginseng is taken 40 minutes before food.

Dose

According to studies:

- On average, 1-3 grams are taken, 40 minutes before meals. In some cases, up to 9 grams are given, however this high of a dose is not needed to see effects.

In my experience:

- Up to 3 grams, no more than twice a day.

Side-effects

Generally considered safe.

- Can cause diarrhea, itching, trouble sleeping, headache, or nervousness.

- Ginseng can increase heart rate, alter blood pressure, cause breast tenderness or induce menstruation. May cause allergic reactions, liver damage, or Stevens-Johnson Syndrome.

- Not recommended during pregnancy.

Mode of Action

- Reduces "uncoupling protein-2". This protein negatively regulates insulin secretion. By reducing this protein ATP levels increase and beta-cell glucose sensing improves.

- Increases insulin production

- Reduces pancreatic cell death (apoptosis) by enhancing beta cell protecting proteins (Bcl-2).

- Increases GLUT4

Triphala

Triphala is one of the most well known Ayurvedic medicines and is quite popular as a remedy for digestive complaints, eye-related disorders, and weight loss. It is often combined with other herbs and used for treating a long list of illnesses – many of which have been scientifically validated through clinical studies. Depending on how you use it, Triphala can be one of the most versatile herbal medicines.

Triphala is a combination of three fruits – Amla (Embelica Officinalis), Vibhitaki (Terminalia Bellerica) and Haritaki (Terminalia Chebula).

Pharmacological properties of each ingredient:

Amla	Vibhitaki	Haritaki
- Anti-diabetic	- Anti-hyperuricemic	- Anti-diabetic
- Hypolipidemic	- Anti-oxidant	- Analgesic
- Anti-bacterial	- Anti-cancer	- Anti-oxidant
- Anti-microbial	- Anti-diarrheal	- Hepatoprotective
- Anti-oxidant	- Anti-microbial	- Anti-viral
- Anti-inflammatory	- Anti-hypertensive	- Anti-inflammatory
- Anti-pyretic	- Hepatoprotective	- Hypolipidemic
- Analgesic	- Anti-pyretic	- Anti-cholesterol
- Adaptogenic	- Anti-ulcerogenic	- Anti-cancer
- Hepatoprotective		- Anti-fungal
- Anti-tumor		- Anti-bacterial
- Anti-ulcerogenic		- Anti-ulcerogenic
- Gastroprotective		- Purgative/Laxative

The uses of Triphala in Ayurvedic medicine include:

- Chronic Fevers
- Piles
- Anal Fistula
- Asthma
- Bronchitis
- Anemia
- Skin Disorders
- Gout
- Edema
- Narcosis
- Obesity
- Ulcers
- Heart Disease (General)
- Anuria
- Diabetes
- Wounds
- Abscesses
- Boils
- Conjunctivitis
- Vision Problems
- Leucorrhea
- Constipation

Clinical evidence supports its use in:

- Diabetes Type 2
- Diabetic Retinopathy
- Gingivitis
- Pre-cancerous Oral Lesions
- Thalassemia
- Periodontal Diseases
- Immature Cataract
- Computer Vision Syndrome
- Increasing Immune Function (NK cells & T-Lymphocytes)

Use in Diabetes

In a placebo-controlled clinical study, patients with Diabetes Type 2 being treated with Triphala experienced significant improvement in blood sugar regulation.

1. The Clinical trial had the following results:

Reduction of:

- Fasting Blood Sugar
- Postprandial Blood Sugar

This was a relatively short study, without assessment of HbA1c. In my experience, Triphala has to be taken long-term in order to make a significant impact. It generally combines very well with Shilajit.

2. One of the ingredients in Triphala is Amla (Mentioned in a Previous Chapter). Clinical studies involving Diabetic patients taking Amla demonstrated a reduction of:

- Fasting Blood Glucose
- Postprandial Blood Sugar
- HbA1c
- Total Cholesterol, LDL-C, Triglycerides (with increase of HDL)
- C-Reactive Protein

Dose

According to studies

- 5 grams, 2 hours after dinner for 45 days. In this study, it was given together with buttermilk

In my experience

- 1 gram, 2-3 times a day, 1 hour before food. While taking Triphala, one should avoid staying up late. My preference is to use Triphala while also supplementing with Shilajit (Discussed in next chapter)

Side-effects

- Generally considered safe.
- May cause diarrhea in larger doses
- Should be avoided in patients with inflammatory bowel disease and other conditions characterized by chronic diarrhea.
- Some patients experience mild gas.
- When correctly used, under an Ayurvedic (BAMS) doctor's supervision and with the appropriate adjuvant, Triphala has no side-effects.

Notes

It is absolutely essential for patients to use Triphala under a doctors supervision as dosing is different for each case. Triphala is one of the most misused Ayurvedic medicines as most websites have information that does not follow the principles of Ayurveda (eg. Time of administration, adjuvants, proportion of each ingredient, etc).

Mode of Action

Inhibits alpha-amylase & alpha-glucosidase. Enhances PPAR-alpha and gamma signaling. Prevents glycation. Given that one of the ingredients is Amla, the mode of action of this fruit is also applicable – see page 30.

Shilajit

Shilajit is the primary option in classical Ayurveda for treating Type 2 Diabetes. The father of surgery, known as "Sushruta", has stated in his book *Sushruta Samhita* (a classical Ayurvedic text), that Shilajit cures a disease known as "Madhu-Meha" which is the Sanskrit/Ayurvedic term for describing what is now known as Diabetes Type 2.

The concept of Madhu-Meha is explained in the chapter on "Ayurvedic perspective on Diabetes".

Shilajit is a Semi-solid exudate that seeps through the rocks of the Himalayan mountains and has been used for thousands of years for treating a wide-range of conditions, predominantly debilitating and metabolic illnesses.

Based on studies, Shilajit appears to have the following pharmacological properties:

- Anti-diabetic
- Anti-oxidant
- Nootropic
- Anti-inflammatory
- Analgesic
- Immunomodulator
- Anti-anxiety
- Anti-ulcer
- Anti-viral
- Spermatogenic
- Aphrodisiac
- Anti-fungal
- Mitochondrial Booster

Its uses in Ayurvedic medicine include:

- Diabetes Type 2
- Sexual Debility
- Edema
- Skin Disease
- CNS disorders
- Asthma
- Obesity
- Anti-aging
- Weakness
- Anemia
- Chronic Bronchitis
- Chronic digestive diseases

Clinical evidence supports its use in:

- Diabetes Type 2
- Infertility
- Low Testosterone
- High Cholesterol
- Function & Regeneration of Skeletal Muscle

Use in Diabetes

In multiple clinical studies, patients with Diabetes Type 2 being treated with Shilajit experienced significant improvement in several aspects of blood sugar regulation as well as blood lipids. Improvement was also seen in various symptoms of Diabetes

Clinical trials had the following results:

Reduction of:

- Fasting Blood Sugar

- Postprandial Blood Sugar
- HbA1c
- Triglycerides & LDL-C
- Diabetes symptoms
    - Polyuria
    - Polydipsia
    - Polyphagia
    - Weakness
    - Burning & Tingling sensation
    - Joint pain
    - Cramps while walking
    - Loss of weight
    - Loss of libido

Increase in

- HDL-C

Dose

According to studies

- 500mg, twice daily with water for 3 months.

In my experience

- 500mg-1000mg, twice a day on an empty stomach. Higher doses (Up to 3000mg) can be used in certain cases, but must be decided upon by an Ayurvedic doctor.

Side-effects

- In the studies analyzed, no adverse drug reactions or side-effects were seen.

- Shilajit should be avoided in Gout or Hyperuricemia.

- In my experience, patients with poor digestive health whom took Shilajit have often experienced gastric discomfort, weight gain, regurgitation of shilajit, indigestion, and in a few cases, gradual or immediate worsening of symptoms. I have also noticed that patients whom use Shilajit brands that are not "Ayurvedic Pharmaceutical companies" often experience signicantly less beneficial results than those whom use the correctly processed and manufactured products.

NOTE:

1. The shilajit used in these studies as well as in standard Ayurvedic treatment is known as **"Shuddha Shilajit"** or **"Purified Shilajit"**. Shilajit must be Ayurvedically processed in order to purify it. As per my inquiries, the regular "Supplements" sold at most health food stores are not processed as it is supposed to be in Ayurveda. Make sure to get the correct type of Shilajit that is produced by an Ayurvedic Pharmaceutical Company. Of course, you need to be careful and make sure the company is one that is GMP certified.

2. Also, shilajit must be used after one has first had their digestion and metabolism corrected as per Ayurvedic standards. Simply believing that you have regular bowel movements and digest food well is not enough to decide whether or not your digestion is proper. Therefore, i strongly advise using purified shilajit under an Ayurvedic doctor's guidance.

Mode of Action

Researchers suggest that shilajit (when used long-term) increases the number of beta-cells in the pancreas and enhances pancreatic function resulting in improved sensitivity of beta-cells as well as improved insulin secretion.

Asanadi Ghana Vati

This is a classical Ayurvedic formulation that is used for several metabolic and skin disorders and has had its efficacy for treating Diabetes validated by clinical studies. It contains 23 ingredients including one of the main sources of Berberine, known as Barberry (Berberis Aristata).

Other ingredients include Pterocarpus Marsupium, Anogeissus Latifolia, Betula Utilis, Calotropis Procera, Sapindus Trifoliatus, Acacia Catechu, Acacia Polyantha, Rubia Cordifolia, Dalbergia Sissoo, Prosopis Specigera, Santalum Album, Pterocarpus Santalinus, Borassus Flabellifer, Butea Monosperma, Aquilaria Agallocha, Grewia Populifolia, Shorea Robusta, Phyllanthus Reticulatas, Anogeissus Latifolia, Holarrhena Antidysenterica, Cassia Fistula and Acacia Leucophloea.

The formulation is mentioned by the Ayurvedic physician known as "Vagbhatta", in his classical Ayurvedic text known as "Ashtanga Hrudaya" - it is located in a part of the book known as Sutra-sthana, chapter 15, verses 19-20.

Based on studies and classical references, this formulation appears to have the following pharmacological properties:

- Anti-diabetic
- Anti-hyperlipidemic
- Anti-oxidant
- Anti-obesity
- Anthelmintic

Its uses in Ayurvedic medicine include:

- Leucoderma
- Leprosy

- Various Skin Diseases
- Intestinal Worms
- Diabetes
- Obesity
- Anemia

Clinical evidence supports its use in:

- Diabetes Type 2
- Hyperlipidemia

Use in Diabetes

In multiple clinical studies, patients with Diabetes Type 2 being treated with Asanadi Gana Vati experienced significant improvement in several aspects of blood sugar regulation as well as blood lipids.

Improvement was also seen in various symptoms of Diabetes.

Clinical trials had the following results:

Reduction of:

- Fasting Blood Sugar
- Postprandial Blood Sugar
- HbA1c
- LDL-C & Triglycerides
- Diabetes symptoms
    - Polyuria
    - Polydipsia
    - Polyphagia
    - Weakness
    - Burning & Tingling sensation
    - Joint pain

- Cramps while walking
- Loss of weight
- Loss of libido

Dose

<u>According to studies:</u>

- 500mg, twice daily, with water for 3 months.

<u>In my experience:</u>

- 500mg, twice daily, with water, before food.

- 5-10 ml of decoction, twice daily, before food.

Side-effects

- No side-effects were seen in the studies.

- Excessive use may result in hypoglycemia.

Mode of Action

Classical Ayurvedic formulas can only be properly understood in terms of Ayurvedic properties:

- Kaphahara -> Reduces kapha dosha
- Sroto-shodana -> Clears the channels
- Kledahara -> Reduces excessive moisture

Ginger

A popular spice and home remedy for a wide-range of disorders, Ginger is quite a versatile spice which has been used in multiple traditional medical systems primarily for nausea, weak digestion, pain and inflammation. Ginger has become so popular for its ability to stop vomiting and nausea that it is now sold as an over-the-counter remedy for morning sickness in pharmacies.

Ginger plays a vital role in digestive and metabolic health and has demonstrated signicant improvement in blood sugar regulation.

Ginger is widely used as part of an Ayurvedic formulation known as "Trikatu", which also contains black pepper and long pepper. This formulation has been used as part of a well-known patented Ayurvedic drug for diabetes, known as "Diabecon".

In studies, Ginger has demonstrated the following pharmacological properties:

- Anti-inflammatory
- Anti-hyperglycemic
- Anti-hyperlipidemic
- Anti-cancer
- Anti-emetic
- Immunomodulator
- Bioavailability Enhancer
- Anti-spasmodic
- Memory Booster
- Fertility Booster
- Testosterone Booster

Uses in Ayurvedic medicine and other traditional medicine systems include:

- Nausea & Vomiting
- Gas
- Abdominal Pain
- Menstrual Cramps
- Headaches
- Poor Appetite
- Cold & Flu
- Arthritis
- Dry Cough
- Piles
- Edema
- Earache
- Fever
- Diarrhea
- Inflammatory Bowel Disease
- Heart Disease

Clinical evidence supports its use in:

- Diabetes Type 2
- High Cholesterol
- Dysmenorrhea
- Morning Sickness
- Chemotherapy-induced Nausea
- Seasickness
- Low Testosterone
- Fertility (Male)
- Osteoarthritis

Use in Diabetes

In multiple clinical studies (including randomized, double-blind, placebo-controlled clinical trials), patients with Diabetes Type 2 being treated with Ginger experienced significant improvement in several aspects of blood sugar regulation

Clinical trials had the following results:

Reduction of:

- Fasting Blood Sugar
- HbA1c

Dose

According to studies

- Up to 3 grams daily for different durations (Between 30-84 days)

In my experience:

- 1 gram, 3 times a day as part of diet. May gradually increase the dose. In some cases I've used up to 10 grams daily for short periods. However, many patients cannot handle such high doses.

Side-effects

The most common side-effect experienced is occasional heartburn. Is known to interact with anti-inflammatories and blood thinners. If using in large doses, check with your doctor and/or pharmacist about possible drug interactions with your current medications.

Mode of Action

Some studies suggest that ginger may directly increase glucose uptake via mechanisms that appear to be independant of insulin – therefore, this may be useful in **Diabetes Type 1** as well. It appears to work via increased GLUT4 translocation. Activities of glucokinase, phosphofructokinase and pyruvate kinase also appear to be increased.

Garlic

Known for its strong flavor, garlic is used all over the world as a very important part of cooking as well as medicine. Garlic is commonly supplemented as:

1. **"Aged garlic extract"** for lowering cholesterol and reducing the length and severity of the flu.

2. **"Lasunadi Vati"**, an Ayurvedic formulation for Rheumatism

Most people are aware of Garlic's benefits for cardiovascular health and fighting off infections, however, several studies have demonstrated its use in Diabetes Type 2 as well.

In studies, Garlic has demonstrated the following pharmacological properties:

- Anti-microbial
- Anti-fungal
- Anti-bacterial
- Anti-viral
- Anti-cancer
- Anti-hyperlipidemic
- Anti-oxidant
- Anti-asthmatic
- Immunomodulator
- Prebiotic
- Anti-mutagenic
- Anti-hypertensive
- Nitric Oxide booster
- Anti-dementia

Use in Ayurvedic medicine and traditional medical systems include:

- Colds
- Heart Disease
- Artherosclerosis
- Skin Diseases & Wounds
- Rheumatoid Arthritis
- Colic
- Splenomegaly
- Asthma
- Epilepsy
- Malarial Fever
- Ear diseases
- Sexual Debility
- Hypertension

Clinical evidence supports its use in:

- Diabetes Type 2
- High Cholesterol
- Hypertension
- Basal Cell Carcinoma
- Common Cold
- Benign Prostate Hyperplasia

Use in Diabetes

In multiple clinical studies (including randomized, double-blind, placebo-controlled clinical trials), patients with Diabetes Type 2 being treated with Garlic experienced significant improvement in several aspects of blood sugar regulation as well as blood lipids

Clinical trials had the following results:

Reduction of:

- Fasting Blood Sugar

- HbA1c
- Fructosamine
- Total Cholesterol
- LDL-C

Dose

According to studies:

- 500mg - 1500mg daily in forms of garlic powder, garlic oil, and aged garlic extract.

In my experience:

- Same as studies, however, I prefer to have patients use it in their food (in quantities of up to 10 grams a day if the patient can handle it). Its best to combine garlic and ginger in food.

I recommend patients to include East Indian foods in their diet as these dishes use large amounts of garlic, ginger and other antihyperglycemic spices.

Majority of the garlic should be added once the heat has been turned off on the stove to avoid losing the organo-sulphur compounds needed for health benefits.

Side-effects

May cause heartburn or the inability to lose the scent of garlic – resulting in bad breath. Garlic may make bleeding disorders worse or interact with blood thinning medications.

- Some people may be allergic to garlic.

- Raw garlic can irritate the digestive tract and cause a burning sensation in the mouth, esophagus and stomach. It can also lead to vomiting and diarrhea.

- If used externally, Garlic can cause severe skin irritation and burns.

- Garlic may possibly interact with several medications – speak to a doctor before using in doses higher than that of regular meals.

Mode of Action

- Appears to increase insulin & C-peptide secretion and release from beta cells.

- Increases the expression of GLUT4 in skeletal muscles.

Mehamudgara Vati

Mehamudgara Vati is a herbo-mineral drug specifically formulated for the treatment of Diabetes as well as several urinary disorders. This formulation is mentioned in the classical Ayurvedic text on mineral-based medicinal preparations known as *Rasendra Chintamani*.

Its ingredients include several well-known anti-diabetic herbs (Including a few mentioned in this book), such as:

- Guggulu *(Commiphora Mukul)*
- Haritaki *(Terminalia Chebula)*
- Bibhitaki *(Terminalia Bellerica)*
- **Amalaki *(Embelica Officinalis)***
- **Ginger**
- Black Pepper
- Long Pepper *(Piper Longum)*
- Trivrut *(Operculina Turpethum)*
- Long Pepper Root
- Bida Lavana *(5 salts)*
- Bilva *(Aegle Marmelos)*
- Gokshura *(Tribulus Terristris)*
- Pomegranate (Bark)
- Devadaru *(Cedrus Deodara)*
- **Barberry *(known source of Berberine)***
- Kiratatikta *(Swertia Chirata)*
- Iron Oxide

This herbs are processed in a **Triphala** Decoction.

Based on its ingredients, studies and traditional uses, Mehamudgara Vati appears to demonstrate the following pharmacological propertics:

- Mucolytic
- Diuretic
- Appetizer
- Anti-pyretic
- Anti-inflammatory
- Anti-oxidant
- Anti-obesity
- Anti-diabetic
- Anti-hyperlipidemic
- Hepatoprotective
- Anti-oxidant
- Immunomodulator
- Anti-stress

Uses in Ayurvedic medicine include:

- Anemia
- Diabetes
- Anorexia
- Poor Appetite
- Indigestion
- Fever
- Dysuria
- Hemorrhagic disorders
- Liver Disorders

Clinical evidence supports its use in:

- Diabetes Type 2

Use in Diabetes

In a clinical study, patients with Diabetes Type 2 being treated with Mehamudgara Vati experienced significant improvement in several aspects of blood sugar regulation as well as blood lipids

Clinical trials had the following results:

Reduction of:

- Fasting Blood Sugar
- Postprandial Blood Sugar

Dose

According to study:

- 750mg, thrice a day after meals for 3 months **(I use the same dose in practice)**

Side-effects

No known side-effects.

- While in clinical practice, this formula is often combined with other antidiabetic drugs, herbs or formulats, such combinations can sometimes lead to low blood sugar if not used under proper supervision of an Ayurvedic doctor.

Mode of Action

Appears to have insulin secretagogue properties & synergistic action when used together with allopathic antidiabetic drugs.

Ayurvedic formulas can only be understood in terms of Ayurvedic properties:

Kleda-Shoshana – Dries up moisture.
Kapha-pitta-shamaka – Reduces kapha and pitta doshas
Kledopayoga – Uses up excess fluid

Phalatrikadi Kwath

Phalatrikadi Kwath is a classical Ayurvedic formulation, specifically formulated for the treatment of urinary disorders and Diabetes Type 2. This formulation is mentioned in the classical Ayurvedic text known as Sharangdhar Sahmita, in a section called "Madhyamkhand", chapter 2, verse 110.

Its ingredients include several well-known anti-diabetic herbs (Including a few mentioned in this book):

- Triphala - *Contains Amla*
- Barberry - *Source of Berberine*
- Musta (Cyperus Rotundus)
- Indravaruni - *Bitter Apple*

Based on its ingredients, studies, and traditional uses, we can infer the following pharmacological properties:

- Anti-diabetic
- Anti-hyperlipidemic
- Anti-inflammatory
- Anti-obesity
- Anti-oxidant
- Mucolytic

Uses in Ayurvedic medicine include:

- Diabetes Type 2
- Urinary Disorders

Clinical evidence supports its use in:

- Diabetes Type 2

Use in Diabetes

In a clinical study, patients with Diabetes Type 2 being treated with Phalatrikadi Kwath together with an Ayurvedic diet and exercise, experienced significant improvement in several aspects of blood sugar regulation.

Clinical trials had the following results:

Reduction of:

- Fasting Blood Sugar
- Postprandial Blood Sugar
- Polyuria

Dose

According to study:

- 50ml, twice daily 1/2 hour before meals, every 12 hours. It is taken together with 1 gram of turmeric and 10ml of honey.

In my experience:

- 50ml – 80ml, twice daily, before meals together with 1 gram of turmeric. Honey or stevia is optional, however is does have a fairly bitter & sour taste. I would recommend not waiting too long to eat after taking this formulation.

Side-effects

In the study, no side effects were experienced.

- In my experience, this formulation can cause low blood sugar when patients consume it together with standard Diabetes drugs.

- This formulation has a pretty strong bitter taste. I have personally tried this formulation and found the taste quite bitter, so I have my patients use either honey or Stevia (Preferably Stevia that does not contain maltodextrin)

Mode of Action

Based on each ingredient:

- Triphala
Inhibits alpha-amylase & alpha-glucosidase. Enhances PPAR-alpha and gamma signaling. Prevents glycation. Given that one of the ingredients is Amla, the mode of action of this fruit is also applicable

- Barberry (Source of Berberine)
Appears to work via induction of glycolysis pathway in cells. Researchers also suggest that barberry may inhibit alpha-glucosidase. Given that the key chemical constituent in Barberry is Berberine, the mode of action of this substance should also be considered (activation of AMPK, etc) – see page 46

- Amla
Based on experimental research, Amla appears to work via regeneration and rejuvenation of the Beta Cells in the pancreas – leading to an increase in insulin production as well as secretion. Amla also contains Chromium, which appears to improve insulin sensitivity.

- Musta
Inhibits alpha-amylase and alpha-glucosidase – thus slowing down the absorption of carbohydrates.

Caper Bush Fruit Extract

Known as "Himsra" in Ayurveda, this herb has demonstrated potent anti-diabetic effects. Recently, it has gotten quite a bit of attention for its ability to reduce ALT and AST liver enzymes along with strong antioxidant properties. Evidence also suggests that it may be used for delaying the signs of aging.

In studies, Caper Bush has demonstrated the following pharmacological properties:

- Anti-oxidant
- Alpha-amylase Inhibitor
- Anti-aging
- Anti-diabetic
- Hepatoprotective
- Anti-cancer
- Anti-bacterial
- Anti-obesity
- Anti-hypertensive
- Anti-microbial
- Anti-hypercholesteremic
- Anti-inflammatory

Uses in Ayurvedic and traditional medical systems include:

- Asthma
- Edema
- Abscess
- Cough
- Fever & Headache
- Liver Disease
- Diabetes
- Sciatica
- Gout

- Skin Diseases
- Hemorrhoids
- Toothache

Clinical evidence supports its use in:

- Diabetes Type 2
- Non-Alcoholic Fatty Liver Disease

Use in Diabetes

In a randomized double-blind, placebo-controlled clinical trial, patients with Diabetes Type 2 being treated with Caper Bush Fruit Extract experienced significant improvement in multiple aspects of blood sugar regulation as well as triglycerides.

Clinical trials had the following results:

Reduction of:

- Fasting Blood Sugar
- HbA1c
- Triglycerides

Dose

According to studies:

- 400mg of caper fruit extract, thrice daily, for two months

In my experience:

- 40-50 grams of caper fruit pickles daily as part of diet.

- I sometimes recommend 50-80ml of a decoction, twice daily.

Side-effects

In the study, there was no hepatotoxicity, nephrotoxicity or any other side effects.

- I have not seen any side-effects in my practice.

- Caper may result in hypoglycemia if combined with other anti-diabetic herbs or a diet deficient in carbohydrates.

Mode of Action

- Appears to inhibit alpha-amylase & hepatic gluconeogenesis. Researchers suggest that beta-cell protection and regeneration may play a role as well.

Bitter Apple

Also known as Bitter Cucumber, Indravaruni and Citrullus Colocynthis, this fruit bearing plant has demonstrated significant anti-diabetic effects in clinical studies. Bitter Apples resemble Watermelons and are quite common in Asia and the Mediterranean Basin with a history of medicinal uses in Arabian traditional medicine and Ayurveda.

Based on studies, Bitter Apple appears to possess the following pharmacological properties:

- Anti-oxidant
- Anti-diabetic
- Anti-lipidemic
- Anti-microbial
- Anti-inflammatory
- Cytotoxic
- Anti-convulsant
- Contraceptive
- Anti-neuropathic

Uses in Ayurvedic medicine and traditional medical systems include:

- Jaundice
- Splenomegaly
- Diabetes
- Bronchitis
- Cleaning of Wounds
- Ascites
- Asthma
- Skin Diseases
- Bloating
- Laxative

- Insect Bites
- Warts
- Alopecia
- Arthritis
- Cervical Adenitis
- Scrotal Enlargement

Clinical evidence supports its use in:

- Diabetes Type 2
- Diabetic Neuropathy
- Hyperlipidemia
- Premature Greying of Hair

Use in Diabetes

In multiple clinical trials (including randomized double-blind, placebo-controlled clinical trials), patients with Diabetes Type 2 being treated with Bitter Apple experienced significant improvement in blood sugar regulation as well as neuropathy.

Clinical trials had the following results:

Reduction of:

- Fasting Blood Sugar
- HbA1c
- Neuropathic Pain

Dose

According to studies:

- 100mg, thrice daily, for 2 months

- 125mg, once daily, before lunch, for 2 months

<u>In my experience:</u>

- 100mg thrice daily, before food.

* In some cases, I have used up to 500mg daily, however, this herb must be used under a doctors supervision as it does have potential side-effects, especially if misused.

Side-effects

- High doses can result in Inflammation of the colon and rectal bleeding.

- Can cause diarrhea, especially when taken multiple times a day.

- Small doses are therapeutic, but high doses are toxic. Bitter Apple is known to be toxic, therefore it must be used under a holistic doctor's supervision.

Mode of Action

In experimental research, Bitter Apple has significantly stimulated the secretion of insulin indicating potent insulinotropic effects. Bitter apple has also demonstrated inhibitory effects on alpha-amylase and alpha-glucosidase.

Milk Thistle (Silymarin)

Known for its active ingredient "Silymarin", this herb is mostly known as a potent liver detoxifier that is backed by multiple clinical studies. Milk Thistle has a 2000+ year long history dating back to the ancient Greeks for the purpose of blood purification and snake bites. Recently, Milk Thistle has also demonstrated significant anti-diabetic potential.

Based on studies, Milk Thistle appears to possess the following pharmacological properties:

- Hepatoprotective
- Anti-inflammatory
- Anti-oxidant
- Anti-fibrotic
- Anti-diabetic
- Hypocholesteremic
- Anti-cancer

Uses in traditional medicine include:

- Cirrhosis
- Hepatitis
- High Cholesterol
- Gall Bladder Disorders
- Jaundice
- Depression
- Skin disorders
- Reduced Milk Flow
- Snake Bites

Clinical evidence supports its use in:

- Non-Alcoholic Fatty Liver Disease

- Acute Hepatitis
- Chronic Hepatitis B
- Acne
- Diabetes Type 2
- Reduced Milk Flow

Use in Diabetes

In multiple clinical trials (including randomized double-blind, placebo-controlled clinical trials), patients with Diabetes Type 2 being treated with Milk Thistle or Silymarin experienced significant improvement in blood sugar regulation.

In one study, Silymarin improved several factors responsible for preventing diabetic nephropathy progression.

Clinical trials had the following results:

Reduction of:

- Fasting Blood Sugar
- HbA1c
- Nephropathy Progression Factors
    - Urinary Albumin Secretion
    - Urinary TNF-a
    - Urinary and serum MDA

Dose

According to studies:

- 200mg - 600mg of Silymarin daily for 45 days to 1 year.

In my experience:

- 1000mg Milk Thistle (whole), 2-3 times daily

- 300mg - 440mg Silymarin daily, in divided doses

Side-effects:

Generally considered safe

- May have mild gastric side-effects such as nausea or mild diarrhea.

- May interact with anti-histamines, anxiolytics, blood thinners and anti-diabetic drugs.

- May interact with chemotherapy drugs.

Mode of Action

- Chemical constituents in Milk Thistle appear to possess peroxisome proliferator-activated receptor γ agonist properties – thus enhancing insulin signaling. Experimental research on non-alcoholic fatty liver disease (a condition often caused by insulin resistance) suggests that Milk Thistle also activates the AMPK pathway.

Management of Diabetic Complications

Diabetic Retinopathy

This is a condition that affects the Eyes and results in degeneration. It develops due to uncontrolled blood sugar damaging the blood vessels going to the light sensitive part of the eye known as the Retina. This results in blurred vision, and in some severe cases, complete vision loss.

There are 2 types:

1. **Non-Proliferative Diabetic Retinopathy**

In this condition, the damaged blood vessels leak fluids and blood and cause the Macula to swell – this is known as Macula Edema - which is the main cause of vision loss. Damage to these blood vessels can also cause them to close off circulation, resulting in Macular Ishcemia. As a result, the Retina is unable to get proper circulation and begins to degenerate.

2. **Proliferative Diabetic Retinopathy**

This is an advanced stage of diabetic eye disease. In this condition, neovascularization (growth of new blood vessels) occurs. These blood vessels then bleed into the eye resulting in floaters or complete vision loss. Eventually, scar tissue develops and this can potentially lead to wrinkling or detachment of the Retina.

Diabetic retinopathy is usually diagnosed with the help of tests such as:

- Fluorescein Angiograpthy
- Optical Coherence Tomography (OCT)

Ayurvedic Solution (Evidence-Based)

Triphala Eye Bath

In Ayurvedic medicine, there is a group of treatment known as "Panchakarma". This basically refers to 5 main treatment and several smaller procedures - one of which is a medicated eye bath – referred to as "Akshi Tarpanam" or "Netra Tarpanam".

This procedure is very simple and not in any way dangerous for the patiient, if done correctly by an Ayurvedic physician (B.A.M.S.) with years of hospital training.

In this procedure, a patient is asked to lay down flat and relax. A bridge is built around the eye using a dough material to create an area to hold the medicine. The eye is then filled with a lipid-based Triphala formulation known as Triphala Ghrita (Read more about Triphala in the previous section). The patient is then kept in that position to relax with their eyes open and bathing in this liquid.

The procedure is repeated for a set number of days, as per the doctor's recommendation.

Evidence:

In a randomized, controlled clinical trial, patients with Non-Proliferative Diabetic Retinopathy whom were treated with Triphala Ghrita Netra Tarpanam as well as given Triphala Ghrita internally, showed significant improvement in visual acuity.

(Reference to the study is in the bibliography)

Triphala has anti-diabetic properties and contains a tannoid principle that appears to inhibit Aldose Reductase – an enzyme that plays a significant role in retinopathy.

Diabetic Neuropathy

Elevated blood sugar can lead to damage of the blood vessels that supply the nerves as well as the nerves themselves – resulting in what is known as Neuropathy. While this most commonly affects the nerves in the hands, feet and legs, it can actually cause damage to other parts of the nervous system as well.

It typically affects the peripheral nerves (sensory and motor), and in some cases, the autonomic nervous system – meaning it can actually affect all major organs and bodily systems.

Neuropathy general starts with cut off blood supply to nerves (Neuronal Ischemia) as well as nerve death due to excess sugar causing damage to the small blood vessels feeding the nerves. In the beginning this leads to the first symptoms of burning, numbness or tinging of the hands and feet.

If left untreated, patients can develop complete loss of feeling and the condition may spread to other parts of the body.

This most commonly occurs in the feet – as a result, patients can become unaware of foot injuries. With reduced circulation, such injuries have a hard time healing due to lack of nutrition, and in severe cases, this condition can lead to tissue death and eventually require amputation.

Symptoms:

- Usually starts with numbness, burning and tingling and hands and feet

As it progresses, it can cause:

- Erectile Dysfunction

- Incontinence
- Inability to Orgasm
- Difficulty swallowing
- Impaired Speech
- Dizziness
- Eyelid Dropping
- Burning Pain
- Dysesthesia
- Retrograde Ejaculation
- Muscle Contractions
- Balance Issues

Diabetic neuropathy is a very broad topic as there are several types and associated syndromes. Hence, it should be treated by a well-versed holistic doctor.

While there are many ways in which this disease can progress, there are a several things that can be done to help in the beginning stages to prevent it from progressing. If your condition is already quite advanced, I suggest going to an Ayurvedic doctor as this requires a very precise treatment protocol.

General Solutions:

1. Guduchyadi Kwath

This is an Ayurvedic medicine which is traditionally used for treating infections, heartburn, gastritis, dysesthesia and burning feet syndrome. It contains Tinospora Cordifolia (Source of Berberine), Coriander, Red Sandalwood, Neem and Wild Himalayan Cherry.

In a randomized open trial, patients were treated with Guduchyadi Kwath and compared to a group taking Vitamin B12 together with Gabapentin. The results showed that Guduchyadi Kwath had equivalent efficacy as the control group except for pain reduction.

To assist with the pain, I often combine Guduchyadi Kwath with the next herb, Bitter Apple.

2. Bitter Apple (Indravaruni)

As mentioned in the section on Bitter Apple, this is a potent anti-diabetic herb with the potential to reduce fasting blood glucose as well as HbA1c. To treat this condition, Bitter Apple extract oil is used topically, daily for several weeks.

In a randomized double-blind placebo-controlled clinical trial, patients with painful diabetic polyneuropathy (PDPN) using bitter apple extract oil for three months, experienced a significant improvement - suggesting that it can decrease pain in patients with PDPN.

3. Atibalamula & Bhumyamalaki

Atibalamula (Abutilon Indicum) is a nervine tonic used in Ayurvedic medicine for treating disorders of the brain and nerves. Bhumyamalaki (Phyllanthus Niruri) is a potent anti-oxidant, anti-inflammatory, hepatoprotective and anti-diabetic herb used for several conditions including liver disorders, diabetes, urinary disorders and burning sensation.

In a clinical study, patients with Diabetic neuropathy were treated with Atibalamula (decoction) and Bhumyamalaki (powder) twice a day for 30 days. Patients experienced a significant reduction in numbness, tingling, burning sensation and pain. The treatment was also able to revert the diminished perception of sensations of vibration, heat and cold.

Other supplements that demonstrated improvement of symptoms in clinical studies:

- **ALA** – Beneficial for several aspects of nerve conduction

- **Benfotiamine** – In multiple clinical studies, it improved symptoms of diabetic neuropathy including pain – <u>I have talked more about this on page 132</u>

- **Micronutrients (Zinc, Vitamin C, E, B1, B2, B6, B12, Biotin, Folic acid, and Magnesium)** – A study stuggests that this combination may improve diabetic neuropathy symptoms

Diabetic Nephropathy

Also known as Diabetic kidney disease, this is a condition in which the kidney's functional units (known as Glomeruli) become damaged due to excess blood sugar. This leads to an increase in the amount of blood passing through the kidneys This extra filtration puts pressure on the kidneys and as a result, they start to leak proteins (Albumin) – this causes what is known as Microalbuminuria.

When <u>small amounts</u> of albumin is excreted in the urine, it is called "microalbuminuria". At this stage, there are several options for treatment and further progression can be prevented or delayed.

When <u>large amounts</u> of albumin is excreted in the urine, it is called "macroalbuminuria". At this point, the condition usually progresses to end-stage renal failure - a very serious condition which requires a patient to either have a kidney transplant or artificial filtration via dialysis.

There are Ayurvedic treatments for renal failure that have been successful in clinical trials

Symptoms

In the intial stages of the disease, patients usually don't experience any signs or symptoms. In the later stages of the disease, patients begin to display the following symptoms:

- High Blood Pressure (That is difficult to control)
- Proteinuria
- Swelling of legs
- Frequent urination (during the day and night)
- Nausea
- Vomiting

- Itchiness of skin
- Loss of appetite
- Headaches
- Fatigue

Hypertensive and Diabetic patients have an increased risk of developing this condition. Other risk factors include a family history of nephropathy and cigarette use.

General Solutions:

1. Tripterygium Wildordii

Also known as "Thunder God Vine", is used in Traditional Chinese medicine for inflammatory and autoimmune conditions. In recent studies, it has shown potential as a method of male birth control as well as a treatment option for diabetic nephropathy.

In a randomized controlled clinical trial, patients taking Tripterygium Wildordii experienced a significant reduction in urine protein levels – demonstrating potential to treat Diabetic nephropathy with proteinuria.

2. Ginkgo Biloba

Known for its potent Adaptogenic and neuro-protective properties, Ginkgo Biloba has become a very popular herb for countering stress and improving neurological health. However, this herb has a long list of benefits including improvement of microalbuminuria.

In multiple randomized clinical trials, patients with Diabetic nephropathy being treated with Ginko Biloba experienced a decrease in urinary albumin excretion rate as well as fasting blood glucose, serum creatinine and blood urea nitrogen.

3. Silymarin

Silymarin, the active chemical constituent of Milk Thistle (a potent liver healing and anti-diabetic herb) has also been used in a randomized, double-blind place-controlled clinical trial and resulted in a reduction in urinary albumin, TNF-a, and MDA.

Ayurvedic Treatment

Ayurvedic treatment for this condition should be managed by an Ayurvedic doctor as the treatment options mentioned are <u>not simple supplements</u> such as those sold at health food stores. **These are classical Ayurvedic medicines that require medical supervision.**

<u>Just for information purposes, these are the Ayurvedic Medicines typically used in published clinical studies:</u>

- Gokshuradi Guggulu, Shilajitvadi Vataka, Punarnavadi Mandura, Bhumyamalaki, Vasa, Guduchi, Bringaraja, and Triphala Guggulu

In published studies, combinations of the above Ayurvedic herbs and formulations were used with much success in reducing microalbuminuria, serum creatinine and blood urea.

Non-Healing Wounds

Due to neuropathy, patients tend to lose sensation in parts of the body such as the lower extremeties. As a result, when they get injured in that area, they may be unaware of it. The problem with neuropathy and blood vessel damage is that blood has a hard time reaching the area of the wound or sore to supply the necessary nutrients needed for healing. This results in slow healing or non-healing ulcers and wounds.

Long term, these wounds can lead to:

- Gangrene
- Fungal Infections
- Bacterial Infections

Once the wound becomes gangrenous, the need for amputation may arise. Therefore, it must be corrected as quickly and efficiently as possible.

Ayurvedic Solutions

1. Neem Oil & Turmeric

Both of these are known for improving skin conditions as well as reducing blood sugar. Neem is used for a wide-range of skin disorders as well as both internal and external ulcers. It is known for its anti-microbial, anti-viral, anti-inflammatory, immune-boosting and wound healing benefits.

Turmeric is also known for it's wound healing, anti-inflammatory, anti-microbial and immune-boosting properties as well as a long history of uses for skin disorders and diabetes.

In a clinical study, the use of Neem oil applied topically and turmeric consumed orally in a dose of 1 gram, thrice daily, were used for treating non-healing wounds. At the end of the study, wound healing along with significant improvement in angiogenesis and DNA concentration were observed.

2. Manuka Honey

Honey is known for its potent anti-microbial properties as well as wound cleansing and healing properties.

In a clinical study, patients with neuropathic diabetic foot ulcers were treated with Manuka honey-impregnated dressings. At the end of the study, there was a significant reduction in healing time as well as rapid disinfection of the foot ulcers.

Honey has also shown promising results when used as an adjuvant for treating gangrene. In fact, it has been used successfully in treating **Fournier's Gangrene** - This is a necrotizing infection that affects the male genitalia – specifically the soft tissue and perineum.

Diabetic Nutrition

Chromium

Chromium is a trace mineral that has become well-known for its role in improving insulin sensitivity. It works by improving the interaction of insulin with cells by increasing insulin receptor phosphoylation as well as increasing insulin binding and insulin receptors.

Chromium works well with patients who have recently developed diabetes type 2 as well as elevated blood sugar due to drugs such as anti-retrovirals.

While many doctors suggest using brewers yeast for getting adequate chromium, I prefer to supplement with Chromium in the Chelate form. You can use chromium under a doctors supervision or consume more Chromium rich foods such as:

- Broccoli
- Grapes
- Potatoes
- Brewers Yeast
- Garlic
- Grass-fed Beef
- Turkey
- Basil

Supplement Dose:

I usually use between 200mcg – 1000mcg. I do not exceed 1000mcg a day.

My preference is to use Chromium Chelate.

Have a holistic physician determine what dose is right for you.

Vanadium

Vanadium is a trace mineral which plays a role in insulin sensitivity in both the liver and muscles. Studies suggest that when used in the form of Vanadyl Sulfate, this mineral can modify certain proteins in the muscles that are involved in insulin signaling. In patients treated with Vanadium, glucose utilization appears to be improved, resulting in lowered fasting blood glucose as well as lowered HbA1c.

While assisting with insulin signaling in Diabetic patients, it does not alter insulin sensitivity in non-diabetic patients – this suggests that it most likely plays a role in some aspect of the pathophysiology of diabetes.

Vanadium-rich foods include Mushrooms, Dill Seeds, Black Pepper, Parsley, and Spinach.

Supplement Dose

Mostly, I use a dose of 10mg daily of vanadyl sulfate. I have used up to 100mg a day with some of my patients/clients. I start with smaller doses of 10mg vanadyl sulfate and then increase it slowly. I do not use 100mg daily for longer than 2-3 weeks. **My recommendation is to use this under a doctors supervision and not to supplement with it on your own.**

Toxicity

There have been links between vanadium and depression. Also, evidence suggests that during manic episodes, there are elevated vanadium levels in the blood. However, in my research, I have come across no solid evidence supporting these connection.

Benfotiamine & Thiamine

Benfotiamine is a fat-soluble synthetic derivative of Thiamine (Vitamin B1). In some parts of the world this nutrient is considered a drug, however, here in the USA it can be purchased as a supplement. It is primarily known for its benefits in diabetic neuropathy and reducing the certain vascular effects of smoking.

In experimental research, Benfotiamine, as well as Thiamine, appear to reduce the mRNA expression of an enzyme known as Aldose Reductase. This enzyme plays a very important role in the pathogenesis of several diabetic complications as it tends to be found in the cornea, retina, lens, kidneys, and myelin sheath (the fatty covering of nerves) – all places where diabetic complications occur.

In various studies, the inhibition of this enzyme has been seen as a therapeutic treatment option for treating/preventing the development of diabetic complications. Benfotiamine especially, is showing much promise in this area.

In clinical studies (including a randomized, double-blind placebo-controlled clinical study), Diabetic patients treated with Thiamine (together with Vitamin B6) or Benfotiamine were able to improve the symptoms of diabetic polyneuropathy including Pain.

Dose

In my experience, due to the fact that I use it in combination with other Ayurvedic medicines, I advise consuming foods rich in B-Vitamins such as Thiamine. With my patients/clients, I do not supplement with Benfotiamine as I have had no need to. However, in studies, Benfotiamine is typically used in doses of 150-900mg daily in divided doses.

Magnesium

Magnesium is well-known for its role in hundreds of processes within the body. One of these processes is that of glucose metabolism and insulin regulation. In fact, multiple studies suggest that low levels of magnesium are linked to the development of insulin resistance and eventually Diabetes Type 2 as well as its complications. The relationship between insulin and magnesium goes both ways as magnesium requires insulin for it to be absorbed into cells as well.

It is a known thing that magnesium is a key co-factor for the mechanism of glucose-transportion into cell membranes and is also responsible for enzymatic actions associated with glucose metabolism. Deficiencies in Magnesium are becoming a common thing along with Vitamin D, therefore I strongly suggest consuming Magnesium rich foods and supplementing with Vitamin D.

In clinical studies (including randomized double-blind placebo-controlled studies) involving patients with Diabetes Type 2 as well as healthy subjects, treatment with magnesium resulted in improvement of blood glucose regulation and insulin sensitivity. Improvements in fasting blood glucose, post-prandial blood glucose, lipid profile, blood pressure and liver enzymes were seen.

Dose

I recommend consuming more magnesium rich foods such as Spinach, Swiss Chard, Avocado, Dark Chocolate, Pumpkin Seeds, Almonds and Black Beans. If supplementing, its best to use Magnesium Chloride, Magnesium Threonate, or Magnesium Malate. In some studies, Magnesium Sulfate has also been used. Dosages vary depending on the patients requirements and current medication, so please use this with a holistic doctor's guidance.

Additional Nutrients

Nutrient Loss & Replenishment

Insulin plays an important role in unlocking cells in order for nutrients to enter. When a patient is "insulin resistant" is means that their cells are not interacting with insulin and as a result, the cells are being starved of certain nutrients. This is how the body composition in such patients changes and results in muscle loss and fat gain.

Some of the nutrients depleted by Diabetes are:

- Potassium
- Zinc
- Vitamin B6
- Vitamin B12
- Antioxidants
- Magnesium
- Vitamin B1

There is also an association between **Vitamin D** deficiencies and the developement of both Diabetes Type 1 & 2. Recent studies also indicate that **Vitamin A** may vital play a role in treating Diabetes Type 1.

With this said, it is important to either supplement or consume foods that are nutrient dense such as Salmon, Kale, Seaweed, Shellfish, Eggs (with Yolks), Liver, Moringa, and Dark chocolate.

If supplementing, do so with a holistic doctor's supervision to ensure proper administration (based on interactions, medications, solubility and several other factors).

Exercise, Yoga, & Pranayama

Exercise

It goes without saying that exercise is beneficial for health, so without going into the general details, I am going to get straight to how it benefits diabetic patients.

Physical activity such as exercise, stimulates skeletal muscle glucose uptake, resulting in lowered blood glucose. Interestingly, this happens independent of insulin. This occurs due to the activity of a glucose transporter known as GLUT4. Physical exercise results in an increase in skeletal muscle GLUT4 expression – which increases glucose uptake. In fact, physical exercise is considered to be the strongest stimulus to increase GLUT4 expression in skeletal muscle.

In simple terms, exercise causes the muscles to absorb glucose from of the blood, regardless of insulin activity.

The best exercises to do would be those that engage multiple muscle groups at once – these are known as compound exercises:

- Squats
- Push-ups
- Bench-Press
- Pull Ups
- Deadlifts
- Overhead Press
- Barbell Row

A more effective way to engage muscles as well as boost the metabolism is to do circuit training. This is where multiple exercises are done in short bursts with short rest periods between each exercise.

The following is an example of a circuit:

- 20 seconds of squats + 10 seconds rest
then
- 20 seconds of push ups + 10 seconds rest
then
- 20 seconds of sit-ups + 10 seconds rest
then
- 20 seconds of pull ups + 1-2 minutes rest

Repeat 5 times.

There are many ways to do circuits. I recommend getting a personal trainer and asking them to put together a routine that involves multiple muscle groups all in the same workout.

The more muscles engaged, the more glucose uptake.

For Diabetic patients, I recommend exercising daily or at least 4 times a week.

Remember to always work within your capacity and don't push yourself too much. Progress is a made over time, not over night.

Yoga

Yoga, at least the physical aspects of it (Asanas), is also effective in lowering blood glucose levels. Of course, this follows the same principle as regular physical exercise in terms of GLUT4 expression in skeletal muscle.

The reason I strongly recommend Yoga Asanas and breathing exercises (pranayama) is the stress reduction and cardiovascular benefits combined with the effect of physical activity on glucose uptake.

Yoga benefits for Diabetes – Clinical Evidence:

In clinical studies, Patients with Diabetes Type 2 whom engaged in Yoga exercise and training experienced a reduction in Fasting blood glucose, Post-prandial blood glucose, HbA1c, and body mass index.

The most effective multi-muscle-group yoga exercise is known as "Surya Namaskar" or "Sun Salutation". This is a series of asanas (poses) that stretch out multiple muscles and apply resistance in a gentle manner.

Pranayama

Pranayama refers to a group of breathing exercises which are traditionally used for calming the mind and treating a wide-range of conditions. These exercise involve controlled breathing such as alternate nostril breathing in which a person breathes in through one nostril and out through the other, then vice versa – this specific breathing exercise is known as Alternate Nostril Breathing or "Nadi Shodhana".

Other breathing exercise include: Ujjay, Sheetali, Kapalbhati, Brahmari, and Omkar – each of these are unique exercises and have different therapeutic benefits.

In clinical studies, Pranayama has been beneficial in multiple conditions including:

- Diabetes
- Hypertension
- Depression
- Asthma
- COPD
- Anxiety

I strongly recommend finding a skilled Yoga teacher and learning to incorporate both Yoga Asanas as well as Pranayama – however, this should be done with the combined assessment of an Ayurvedic doctor as the use of each exercise is based on the underlying illness.

I have met many Yoga practitioners and teachers who claim to "know Ayurveda", however, it takes **years of clinical training in an Ayurvedic medical school** to truly understand Ayurveda, therefore any "Ayurvedic" assessment should only be done by an Ayurvedic doctor holding the "BAMS" degree.

Dietary Advice

What is most effective?

As a general rule, Diabetic patients are often advised to consume foods that have a low "glycemic index" or "glycemic load", but what exactly does that mean? Before getting into what diet works best for Diabetes, lets talk about this idea of glycemic load and index, just in case you don't wish to follow the diet.

Glycemic Index (GI)

This is a measurement of the quality of a carbohydrate and the effect it will have on blood glucose levels. It is measured in values ranging from 0 to 100.

Foods with a low glycemic index (<55) digest and absorb slower, resulting in a lower and more gradual rise in blood sugar. By consuming foods in this range, it is easier to manage blood glucose levels and reduce the need for insulin. These foods tend to also keep a person satisfied for longer due to their slow digestion.

High glycemic index foods (70>) result in quick and high rises in blood glucose levels. As a general rule, this should be avoided as much as possible when trying to manage diabetes while medium GI foods (56-69) can be used in moderation.

How can you know the Glycemic Index of a food?

Below is a list of common carbohydrate rich foods and their glycemic indexes. There are many online sources for figuring out the glycemic index of food – you can literally just search for most of them online.

Low GI	Medium GI	High GI
Apples	Mango	Dates
Bananas	Papaya	Watermelon
Blueberries	Cantaloupe	Kiwi
Cherries	Apricot	Grapes
Coconut	Pineapple	Pumpkin
Cranberries	Peaches	Potato
Beans (General)	Raisins	Parsnips
Oranges	Noodles	French Fries
Strawberries	Bulgur	Bagels
Asparagus	Oatmeal (rolled)	Most Packaged Cereals
Almonds	Pita Bread	French Baguette
Brussel Sprouts	Rye	Gnocchi
Cabbage	Wild Rice	Muesli
Carrots	Mayo	White Pita Bread
Cucumber	Black-eyed peas	White Rice
Eggplant	Ketchup	Puffed Rice
Celery	Mustard	Rice Pasta
Kale	Nutella	Rice Cakes
Lettuce	Chestnuts	White Bread
Okra	Whole Wheat	Ice Cream
Peppers	Basmati Rice	Canned Lentils
Pickles	Quick Oats & Porridge	Canned Kidney Beans
Tomatoes	Bran Muffins	Corn Syrup
Spinach	Linguine	Donuts

Zucchini	Sweet Potato	Croissants
Barley	Green Peas	Popcorn
Chickpeas & Hummus		Cookies (General Packaged)
Quinoa		White Sugar
Rice Bran		Pizza (Wheat)
Plain Yogurt		High Fructose Corn Syrup

Glycemic Load

This is an overall measurement of the glycemic index together with the quantity of carbohydrates in a food. Obviously, this also plays a significant role in the rate and level of rise in blood sugar.

It is calculated by multiplying the glycemic index (as a percentage) by the amount of carbohydrates (grams) in a food.

Eg. A medium apple has a GI of 40, with about 25 grams of carbohydrates.

So, 25 x 40% = 10.

Therefore, the glycemic load for a medium apple is 10. This is considered a low glycemic load.

Low Glycemic Load = 10 or less
Medium Glycemic Load = 11-19
High Glycemic Load = 20 or more

Lower glycemic load foods are going to result in lower rises in blood sugar levels.

I personally recommend following glycemic index more than glycemic load.

However, there is a diet that if followed correctly, doesn't require you to know anything about glycemic index or load and is what appears to work quite well in most people who I've helped with managing Diabetes.

Based on my research and experience, it is my belief that the best diet for controlling diabetes and blood sugar levels in general, is the **Ketogenic Diet**. While this diet is not suitable for absolutely everyone, it certainly does appear to work in the majority of people.

I usually don't recommend people to get their information from the internet, however, I strongly suggest researching the Ketogenic diet and its results before dismissing this idea.

What is the Ketogenic Diet?

The Ketogenic diet is basically a diet that involves a high amount of fat, very little or no carbs and an adequate amount of protein.

Yes, you read that right. "High amount of fat", and NO it won't cause you to gain fat or have a heart attack if done right with a doctors guidance. The clogging of arteries requires a lot more than fat in your diet and is actually appearing to be more related to inflammatory activities.

The goal of this diet is to put the body into a state where it burns fats for fuel rather than relying on carbohydrates and glucose – this is known as Ketosis (Do not confused with diabetic ketosis).

Ketosis is basically a state in which the liver breaks down fat into fatty acids and glycerol. The fatty acids are further broken down into Ketones, which effectively work as energy providing substances. The body is able to run off of these ketones quite efficiently, however, it does take a little "getting used to", so in the beginning you may have a few mild side-effects such as the "Keto flu".

In a multiple studies, patients with Diabetes Type 2 whom followed a low carbohydrate ketogenic diet experienced improved glycemic control. The ketogenic diet even outperformed the conventional low calorie diet in obese diabetic patients.

So how do you do this diet?

Basically, you need to get about 80% of your calories from fat and the rest from protein and a few carbohydrates. Aim for less than 50 grams of carbs a day.

Fat rich foods:
- Avocado
- Ghee
- Olive Oil
- Grass-fed butter
- Coconut Oil
- Eggs
- Nuts, Seeds (especially Chia Seeds)
- Plain Greek Yogurt

Protein Sources:
- Grass-fed beef
- Lamb
- Salmon
- Chicken (preferably Chicken Thighs)
- Organ Meats (Liver, Kidneys, Heart)
- Trotters
- Eggs
- Seafood
- Dairy (A2 – Look up A2 milk)
- Mung Beans
- Seitan
- Tempeh
- Tofu

Carbohydrate Foods that are suitable:
- Cauliflower
- Broccoli
- Brussel Sprouts
- Kale
- Cabbage
- Spinach
- Lettuce
- Swiss Chard
- Asparagus
- Cucumber
- Zucchini

There are a wide range of foods that are keto-friendly.

It is crucial to avoid all sugars, sodas, cakes, candy, cookies, pastries, and other carbohydrate rich foods. There are plenty of keto recipes online, even for making keto-bread and cauliflower pizza. Foods such as noodles and rice can be replaced with zucchini noodles and cauliflower rice.

For the purpose of weight loss, calorie counting is not always needed. However, for controlling blood sugar, one should still not go overboard. Remember that proteins can also trigger a sugar spike if too much is consumed.

NOTE: When combining anti-diabetic foods and herbs together with a ketogenic diet, careful monitoring of blood sugar is essential to avoid hypoglycemia. With that said, it is absolutely essential to follow this under a holistic doctor's supervision. Do not underestimate the potency of the herbs, foods, nutrients and formulations mentioned in this book combined with a ketogenic diet in lowering blood sugar levels.

Diabetes Type 1

The management of Diabetes Type 1 starts with the use the insulinotropic and insulin mimetic foods and herbs. Insulinotropics are substances that support the release of insulin from the pancreas. Insulin mimetics mimic the activity of insulin itself. By supporting the production of endogenous insulin or providing insulin-like compounds through diet, we can potentially reduce the need for injecting insulin.

Of course, this is only one part of the problem. The other problem is the presence of antibodies. While the reduction of antibodies is something I have seen in practice, the methodology used for achieving this has not yet been used in clinical studies, and this book is strictly evidence-based. I will however, publish my own case studies on my website in the near future, along with the specifics of my protocols for reducing the antibodies.

Insulinotropic & Insulin Mimetic Foods & Herbs

Gymnema Sylvestre – known as the sugar destroyer, this herb contains "Gymnemic acid" which appears to be insulinotropic in nature as it improves blood sugar levels and enhance endogenous insulin in patients with type 1 diabetes. It has a history of over 5000 years of use in classical Ayurveda and has been used in clinical studies for treating Diabetes Type 1 & 2. In experimental research, Gymnema Sylvestre has demonstrated potential to regenerate the insulin-secreting beta cells located in the pancreas.

You can find more information on how to use this herb on **page 31**

Bitter Melon – this is typically used in traditional medicine as well as Ayurveda for improving insulin sensitivity and contains a chemical known as "polypeptide-k" that appears to be very similar in nature to that of insulin itself. In experimental research, an extract of bitter melon has demonstrated both insulin secretagogue and insulin mimetic activity. In clinical research, bitter melon has had anti-hyperglycemic effects in patients with Diabetes. As per my research, it has not yet been used in clinical trials for Type 1, however, in my experience it has been quite useful (especially in newly diagnosed cases) when combined with Fenugreek.

Fenugreek – has a history of being able to support hormone production in the body. It's been used as a home remedy for high blood sugar in India for many years and with much success. In clinical studies, Fenugreek has been effective in reducing blood glucose and urinary glucose levels significantly in patients with Diabetes Type 1. As mentioned in the previous paragraph, I have witnessed quite impressive results when combined with Bitter melon.

Other Foods/Herbs that appear to have insulin-secretagogue or insulin-mimetic properties in experimental studies are:

- Garlic, Ginger, Flax Seeds, Aloe Vera,
- Loquat, Java Plum, Guava, Bitter Apple
- Caper Bush Fruit Extract
- Panax Ginseng & American Ginseng
- Heal-All, Jackfruit Leaf, Walnut Leaf
- Kanchanar
- Shilajit, Withania Coagulans, Chinese Licorice
- Mehamudgara Vati
- Spanish Sage
- Nettle

Yoga Exercise for Massaging the Pancreas

Think of the Pancreas as a muscle that has become fatigued. Much like how prolonged sessions of writing or playing the piano can fatigue the muscles in your forearm. Massaging that forearm, helps restore circulation and enables it to function better. Similarly, the Pancreas can also receive better circulation by doing exercises or massaging that region.

(Please keep in mind that you should be on a strict anti-inflammatory diet before doing this exercise)
In my practice, patients/clients are advised to massage the Pancreas by performing a Yogic exercise known as **"Agni-sar Kriya"**

This Yogic practice is performed by moving the abdominal muscles in and out and continuous manner.

Proper guidance is required for performing this exercise so that it is properly done.

Here are the steps for performing this Yogic Practice:
Step 1. Sit in a comfortable position and make sure that your back is straight.
Step 2. Maintain proper breathing, be relaxed and calm.
Step 3. Now, exhale completely and while maintaining this state of not having your lungs filled, begin the next step
Step 4. Gently pull your belly in (as if trying to make your naval touch your spine) and relax, then pull your belly in again, then relax (do this continuously for a few seconds.
Step 5. Then release, relax and breathe normally for a few seconds.

Continue breathing normally for a while and then repeat.
Continue this 5-6 times at first. Afterwards, you may extend the length of practice.

Make sure that you do not strain or apply pressure on anything while performing this. It is meant to be gentle and relaxed.

There are many instructional videos on YouTube for this practice, yet i strongly advise professional guidance.

Contraindications for this practice include but are not limited to: Blood pressure problems, abdominal hernia, injuries to the abdominal area, severe anemia, asthma, gastritis and other inflammatory conditions of the gastrointestinal tract, diarrhea, and GERD.

How does this practice work?

Basically, by moving the abdominal muscles in and out (without the air pressure getting in the way), you are directly compressing and releasing the abdominal organs including the pancreas. Thus increasing circulation to the area which provides it with better nourishment.

* *Another method of massaging the Pancreas is by performing an abdominal massage. Gently massage the abdominal region in a clock-wise direction. Do this daily to increase circulation in the area – It is best to use a medicated oil for this such as classically prepared Ashwagandha Oil. Of course, like with any other topical substance, oils should be first tested for any reactions by applying a small amount to the skin and waiting at least 2 hours to see if any allergic reaction occurs. Other oils may be used as well (as per an Ayurvedic doctors advice).*

Milk & Diabetes Type 1

Specifically A1 milk, appears to be quite a problem for Diabetes type 1. It contains a protein known as A1- Beta-Casein which appears to have a negative impact on various aspects of health. While the studies are not conclusive, the consumption of A1 milk by children has been linked (in multiple studies) to an increased risk of developing Diabetes Type 1.

The milk debate has been going on for years now, however in my experience, A2 milk has had less of a inflammatory response in my clients/patients. More so, my patients in Dubai, South Africa, India, and European countries have all confirmed that by switching to A2 milk, they were able to avoid many of the unwanted effects of drinking regular store-bought A1 milk (such as Diarrhea, Bloating, Congestion, etc).

I usually don't support the consumption of milk at all as most milk these days is terrible quality A1 milk from chronically stressed cows that are pumped with hormones and fed grains. However, in my experience, organic high quality A2 milk from countries other than the USA tends to react much better with my clients/patients as well as myself.

<u>Other inflammatory/unhealthy foods that should be avoided in autoimmune conditions:</u>

- Soy
- Corn
- Wheat

- Barley
- Oats
- Processed Meats & processed foods in general
- White Sugar
- Dairy (more so A1)
- Vegetable Oils
- Refined Carbohydrates
- Alcohol
- Soda
- Packaged Foods and candy
- Fried Foods

Conclusion

Considering the fact that in the USA, the average Diabetic spends over $13,000 a year in medical costs, you will find that the supplements, herbs and formulations mentioned in this book are ridiculously cost effective.

Approximately eight months ago, a close relative of mine was diagnosed with Diabetes and immediately put on treatment which resulted in an average monthly expense of $700. After approaching me for treatment, I put them on a protocol including only three of the options mentioned in this book, resulting in a monthly expense of only $29. After six months, they no longer needed any herbal medicines and are now able to manage their condition fairly easily with diet, exercise and herbs they grow at home.

I personally find it quite unfair that any sick person should have to pay such ridiculous prices for medicines that they will be forced to consume for the rest of their life.

I find it shocking that patients are completely unaware that there are foods and spices in their kitchens that have demonstrated the potential to effectively manage this condition in clinical studies. Shouldn't their doctors inform them?

This is why I wrote this book – to inform the world of cheaper natural options available to them. Ignorance is a heavy price to pay, especially when it results in people creating debts just to stay alive while literally remaining sick and getting worse with time.

Finding a supportive physician

As you may have noticed, I have mentioned several times in this book that in order to get safe and effective results, you must have the guidance of an experienced holistic physician, preferably an Ayurvedic physician.

A holistic physician with good training should be aware of several of the options mentioned in this book except the Ayurvedic formulations.

Ayurvedic medicines are administered according to Ayurvedic medical principles of treatment and therefore, an Ayurvedic doctor will be needed.

How to find an Ayurvedic doctor

This presents much difficulty as here in the USA many people call themselves Ayurvedic "specialists", "masters", "practitioners" and so many other titles, without actual Ayurvedic <u>medical</u> training. Some of these practitioners claim to be taught by gurus and so-called masters.

Let me be frank, in the USA there is <u>no regulation</u> of Ayurvedic Medicine and as a result, <u>there is no actual American "medical" degree for Ayurveda</u> that involves the standard 5 & 1/2 to 6 years of hospital training along with providing a medical license of any sort.

However, outside of the USA, there is an actual medical degree in Ayurveda that is recognized in multiple countries and grants one an <u>actual medical license</u> in those countries - that is the five and a half to six year long **Bachelor's of Ayurvedic Medicine & Surgery (BAMS) degree.**

While BAMS is not yet recognized in the USA, it is an authentic <u>Ayurvedic medical degree</u> that involves years of clinical training (in a hospital) as well as a medical internship. This degree involves attending classes six days a week for approximately six years including practical hospital training for the entire duration.

The next best thing is to visit a "Certified Ayurvedic Practitioner". An Ayurvedic Practitioner generally receives an education that provides them with the skills needed to advise you about many of the options mentioned in this book. They do not possess the same training as a BAMS Ayurvedic doctor but they do have an Ayurvedic education that is enough to provide you with the guidance you need.

If you are seeking Ayurvedic treatment, my recommendation is to find someone with either of these qualifications. It doesn't matter if the person is an MD, ND, DC, or any other type of physician. If they do not have BAMS or are a Certified Ayurvedic Practitioner, they do not have the same training as me and I cannot recommend you to seek Ayurvedic advice from them.

Here in the USA, due to the lack of licensing and regulation, a person can call themselves an Ayurvedic specialist, master, king or even God if they wish. <u>If you want authentic Ayurvedic treatment, the only credible option is to find an Ayurvedic doctor holding the B.A.M.S. Degree or an Ayurvedic Practitioner that is board-certified with the National Ayurvedic Medical Association (NAMA).</u>

It is not my goal to talk down about other "practitioners" but to inform the public of the facts. It is the responsible thing for me to do considering that I have put so much information in your hands that you will need proper guidance with.

As a man who believes in authenticity, I will always stand for what I believe to be true and effective, especially for those who come to me for help. The fact that you have read this book means that you are seeking help, and it is my duty to lead you down the right path.

Bibliography

Role of stress

Chronic Stress

1. Yan YX, Xiao HB, Wang SS, Zhao J, He Y, Wang W, Dong J. Investigation of the Relationship Between Chronic Stress and Insulin Resistance in a Chinese Population. J Epidemiol. 2016 Jul 5;26(7):355-60. doi: 10.2188/jea.JE20150183. Epub 2016 Jan 30. PubMed PMID: 26830350; PubMed Central PMCID: PMC4919480.

Interleukin-6

1. Kim JH, Bachmann RA, Chen J. Interleukin-6 and insulin resistance. Vitam Horm. 2009;80:613-33. doi: 10.1016/S0083-6729(08)00621-3. Review. PubMed PMID: 19251052.

2. Hoene M, Weigert C. The role of interleukin-6 in insulin resistance, body fat distribution and energy balance. Obes Rev. 2008 Jan;9(1):20-9. Epub 2007 Oct 23. Review. PubMed PMID: 17956545.

3. Senn JJ, Klover PJ, Nowak IA, Mooney RA. Interleukin-6 induces cellular insulin resistance in hepatocytes. Diabetes. 2002 Dec;51(12):3391-9. PubMed PMID: 12453891.

Catecholamines

1. Barth E, Albuszies G, Baumgart K, Matejovic M, Wachter U, Vogt J, Radermacher P, Calzia E. Glucose metabolism and catecholamines. Crit Care Med. 2007 Sep;35(9 Suppl):S508-18. Review. PubMed PMID: 17713401.

Cortisol

1. Jeong IK. The role of cortisol in the pathogenesis of the metabolic syndrome. Diabetes Metab J. 2012 Jun;36(3):207-10. doi: 10.4093/dmj.2012.36.3.207. Epub 2012 Jun 14. PubMed PMID: 22737660; PubMed Central PMCID: PMC3380124.

2. Adam TC, Hasson RE, Ventura EE, Toledo-Corral C, Le KA,

Mahurkar S, Lane CJ, Weigensberg MJ, Goran MI. Cortisol is negatively associated with insulin sensitivity in overweight Latino youth. J Clin Endocrinol Metab. 2010 Oct;95(10):4729-35. doi: 10.1210/jc.2010-0322. Epub 2010 Jul 21. PubMed PMID: 20660036; PubMed Central PMCID: PMC3050109.

3. Holmäng A, Björntorp P. The effects of cortisol on insulin sensitivity in muscle. Acta Physiol Scand. 1992 Apr;144(4):425-31. PubMed PMID: 1605044.

Herbal Medicines

Sage

1. Sajjadi F, Baghbanian P, Asgari S, Naderi GA, Alikhasi H, Mohammadi Fard N. et al. The effect of hydroalcoholic extract of Salvia officinal on diabetic patients. J Res Med Sci. 2003;4:318–24.

2. Kianbakht S, Nabati F, Abasi B. Salvia officinalis (Sage) Leaf Extract as Add-on to Statin Therapy in Hypercholesterolemic Type 2 Diabetic Patients: a Randomized Clinical Trial. Int J Mol Cell Med. 2016 Summer;5(3):141-148. Epub 2016 Sep 3. PubMed PMID: 27942500; PubMed Central PMCID: PMC5125366.

3. Kianbakht S, Dabaghian FH. Improved glycemic control and lipid profile in hyperlipidemic type 2 diabetic patients consuming Salvia officinalis L. leaf extract: a randomized placebo. Controlled clinical trial. Complement Ther Med. 2013 Oct;21(5):441-6. doi: 10.1016/j.ctim.2013.07.004. Epub 2013 Aug 6. PubMed PMID: 24050577.

Amla

1. Akhtar MS, Ramzan A, Ali A, Ahmad M. Effect of Amla fruit (Emblica officinalis Gaertn.) on blood glucose and lipid profile of normal subjects and type 2 diabetic patients. Int J Food Sci Nutr. 2011 Sep;62(6):609-16. doi: 10.3109/09637486.2011.560565. Epub 2011 Apr 18. PubMed PMID: 21495900

2. Chen TS, Liou SY, Wu HC, Tsai FJ, Tsai CH, Huang CY,

Chang YL. Efficacy of epigallocatechin-3-gallate and Amla (Emblica officinalis) extract for the treatment of diabetic-uremic patients. J Med Food. 2011 Jul-Aug;14(7-8):718-23. doi: 10.1089/jmf.2010.1195. Epub 2011 Jun 1. PubMed PMID: 21631363

3. D'souza JJ, D'souza PP, Fazal F, Kumar A, Bhat HP, Baliga MS. Anti-diabetic effects of the Indian indigenous fruit Emblica officinalis Gaertn: active constituents and modes of action. Food Funct. 2014 Apr;5(4):635-44. doi: 10.1039/c3fo60366k. Review. PubMed PMID: 24577384.

4. Usharani P, Fatima N, Muralidhar N. Effects of Phyllanthus emblica extract on endothelial dysfunction and biomarkers of oxidative stress in patients with type 2 diabetes mellitus: a randomized, double-blind, controlled study. Diabetes Metab Syndr Obes. 2013 Jul 26;6:275-84. doi: 10.2147/DMSO.S46341. Print 2013. PubMed PMID: 23935377; PubMed Central PMCID: PMC3735284.

Gymnema

1. Kumar SN, Mani UV, Mani I. An open label study on the supplementation of Gymnema sylvestre in type 2 diabetics. J Diet Suppl. 2010 Sep;7(3):273-82. doi: 10.3109/19390211.2010.505901. PubMed PMID: 22432517

2. Baskaran K, Kizar Ahamath B, Radha Shanmugasundaram K, Shanmugasundaram ER. Antidiabetic effect of a leaf extract from Gymnema sylvestre in non-insulin-dependent diabetes mellitus patients. J Ethnopharmacol. 1990 Oct;30(3):295-300. PubMed PMID: 2259217.

3. Shanmugasundaram ER, Rajeswari G, Baskaran K, Rajesh Kumar BR, Radha Shanmugasundaram K, Kizar Ahmath B. Use of Gymnema sylvestre leaf extract in the control of blood glucose in insulin-dependent diabetes mellitus. J Ethnopharmacol. 1990 Oct;30(3):281-94. PubMed PMID: 2259216

4. Kurian GA, Manjusha V, Nair SS, Varghese T, Padikkala J. Short-term effect of G-400, polyherbal formulation in the

management of hyperglycemia and hyperlipidemia conditions in patients with type 2 diabetes mellitus. Nutrition. 2014 Oct;30(10):1158-64. doi: 10.1016/j.nut.2014.02.026. Epub 2014 Mar 14. PubMed PMID: 24976431.

Cinnamon

1. Beejmohun V, Peytavy-Izard M, Mignon C, Muscente-Paque D, Deplanque X, Ripoll C, Chapal N. Acute effect of Ceylon cinnamon extract on postprandial glycemia: alpha-amylase inhibition, starch tolerance test in rats, and randomized crossover clinical trial in healthy volunteers. BMC Complement Altern Med. 2014 Sep 23;14:351. doi: 10.1186/1472-6882-14-351. PubMed PMID: 25249234; PubMed Central PMCID: PMC4246455.

2. Lu T, Sheng H, Wu J, Cheng Y, Zhu J, Chen Y. Cinnamon extract improves fasting blood glucose and glycosylated hemoglobin level in Chinese patients with type 2 diabetes. Nutr Res. 2012 Jun;32(6):408-12. doi: 10.1016/j.nutres.2012.05.003. Epub 2012 Jun 14. PubMed PMID: 22749176.

3. Hlebowicz J, Darwiche G, Björgell O, Almér LO. Effect of cinnamon on postprandial blood glucose, gastric emptying, and satiety in healthy subjects. Am J Clin Nutr. 2007 Jun;85(6):1552-6. PubMed PMID: 17556692.

4. Khan A, Safdar M, Ali Khan MM, Khattak KN, Anderson RA. Cinnamon improves glucose and lipids of people with type 2 diabetes. Diabetes Care. 2003 Dec;26(12):3215-8. PubMed PMID: 14633804

Vinegar

1. Johnston CS, Gaas CA. Vinegar: medicinal uses and antiglycemic effect. MedGenMed. 2006 May 30;8(2):61. Review. PubMed PMID: 16926800; PubMed Central PMCID: PMC1785201.

2. Ostman E, Granfeldt Y, Persson L, Björck I. Vinegar supplementation lowers glucose and insulin responses and increases satiety after a bread meal in healthy subjects. Eur J Clin

Nutr. 2005 Sep;59(9):983-8. PubMed PMID: 16015276.

3. Johnston CS, Kim CM, Buller AJ. Vinegar improves insulin sensitivity to a high-carbohydrate meal in subjects with insulin resistance or type 2 diabetes. Diabetes Care. 2004 Jan;27(1):281-2. PubMed PMID: 14694010.

Salacia

1. Hao L, Schlussel Y, Fieselmann K, Schneider SH, Shapses SA. Appetite and Gut Hormones Response to a Putative α-Glucosidase Inhibitor, Salacia Chinensis, in Overweight/Obese Adults: A Double Blind Randomized Controlled Trial. Nutrients. 2017 Aug 12;9(8). pii: E869. doi: 10.3390/nu9080869. PubMed PMID: 28805670; PubMed Central PMCID: PMC5579662.

2. Jeykodi S, Deshpande J, Juturu V. Salacia Extract Improves Postprandial Glucose and Insulin Response: A Randomized Double-Blind, Placebo Controlled, Crossover Study in Healthy Volunteers. J Diabetes Res. 2016;2016:7971831. Epub 2016 Oct 10. PubMed PMID: 27803937; PubMed Central PMCID: PMC5075619.

3. Koteshwar P, Raveendra KR, Allan JJ, Goudar KS, Venkateshwarlu K, Agarwal A. Effect of NR-Salacia on postprandial hyperglycemia: A randomized double blind, placebo-controlled, crossover study in healthy volunteers. Pharmacogn Mag. 2013 Oct;9(36):344-9. doi: 10.4103/0973-1296.117831. PubMed PMID: 24124287; PubMed Central PMCID: PMC3793340.

4. Williams JA, Choe YS, Noss MJ, Baumgartner CJ, Mustad VA. Extract of Salacia oblonga lowers acute glycemia in patients with type 2 diabetes. Am J Clin Nutr. 2007 Jul;86(1):124-30. PubMed PMID: 17616771.

Fraxinus Excelsior

1. Zulet MA, Navas-Carretero S, Lara y Sánchez D, Abete I, Flanagan J, Issaly N, Fança-Berthon P, Bily A, Roller M, Martinez JA. A Fraxinus excelsior L. seeds/fruits extract benefits glucose

homeostasis and adiposity related markers in elderly overweight/obese subjects: a longitudinal, randomized, crossover, double-blind, placebo-controlled nutritional intervention study. Phytomedicine. 2014 Sep 15;21(10):1162-9. doi: 10.1016/j.phymed.2014.04.027. Epub 2014 May 28. PubMed PMID: 24877717.

2. Visen P, Saraswat B, Visen A, Roller M, Bily A, Mermet C, He K, Bai N, Lemaire B, Lafay S, Ibarra A. Acute effects of Fraxinus excelsior L. seed extract on postprandial glycemia and insulin secretion on healthy volunteers. J Ethnopharmacol. 2009 Nov 12;126(2):226-32. doi: 10.1016/j.jep.2009.08.039. Epub 2009 Aug 31. PubMed PMID: 19723572.

Berberine

1. Pérez-Rubio KG, González-Ortiz M, Martínez-Abundis E, Robles-Cervantes JA, Espinel-Bermúdez MC. Effect of berberine administration on metabolic syndrome, insulin sensitivity, and insulin secretion. Metab Syndr Relat Disord. 2013 Oct;11(5):366-9. doi: 10.1089/met.2012.0183. Epub 2013 Jun 28. PubMed PMID: 23808999.

2. Dong H, Wang N, Zhao L, Lu F. Berberine in the treatment of type 2 diabetes mellitus: a systemic review and meta-analysis. Evid Based Complement Alternat Med. 2012;2012:591654. doi: 10.1155/2012/591654. Epub 2012 Oct 15. PubMed PMID: 23118793; PubMed Central PMCID: PMC3478874.

3. Yin J, Xing H, Ye J. Efficacy of berberine in patients with type 2 diabetes mellitus. Metabolism. 2008 May;57(5):712-7. doi: 10.1016/j.metabol.2008.01.013. PubMed PMID: 18442638; PubMed Central PMCID: PMC2410097.

Nigella Sativa

1. Daryabeygi-Khotbehsara R, Golzarand M, Ghaffari MP, Djafarian K. Nigella sativa improves glucose homeostasis and serum lipids in type 2 diabetes: A systematic review and meta-analysis. Complement Ther Med. 2017 Dec;35:6-13. doi: 10.1016/j.ctim.2017.08.016. Epub 2017 Aug 30. Review. PubMed

PMID: 29154069.

2. Heshmati J, Namazi N. Effects of black seed (Nigella sativa) on metabolic parameters in diabetes mellitus: a systematic review.Complement Ther Med. 2015 Apr;23(2):275-82. doi: 10.1016/j.ctim.2015.01.013. Epub 2015 Feb 9. Review. PubMed PMID: 25847566.

3. Kaatabi H, Bamosa AO, Badar A, Al-Elq A, Abou-Hozaifa B, Lebda F, Al-Khadra A, Al-Almaie S. Nigella sativa improves glycemic control and ameliorates oxidative stress in patients with type 2 diabetes mellitus: placebo controlled participant blinded clinical trial.PLoS One. 2015 Feb 23;10(2):e0113486. doi: 10.1371/journal.pone.0113486. eCollection 2015. PubMed PMID: 25706772; PubMed Central PMCID: PMC4338020.

4. Kaatabi H, Bamosa AO, Lebda FM, Al Elq AH, Al-Sultan AI. Favorable impact of Nigella sativa seeds on lipid profile in type 2 diabetic patients. J Family Community Med. 2012 Sep;19(3):155-61. doi: 10.4103/2230-8229.102311. PubMed PMID: 23230380; PubMed Central PMCID: PMC3515953.

5. Najmi A, Nasiruddin M, Khan RA, Haque SF. Effect of Nigella sativa oil on various clinical and biochemical parameters of insulin resistance syndrome. Int J Diabetes Dev Ctries. 2008 Jan;28(1):11-4. doi: 10.4103/0973-3930.41980. PubMed PMID: 19902033; PubMed Central PMCID: PMC2772004.

Nettle

1. Kianbakht S, Khalighi-Sigaroodi F, Dabaghian FH. Improved glycemic control in patients with advanced type 2 diabetes mellitus taking Urtica dioica leaf extract: a randomized double-blind placebo-controlled clinical trial. Clin Lab. 2013;59(9-10):1071-6. PubMed PMID: 24273930.

2. Namazi N, Tarighat A, Bahrami A. The effect of hydro alcoholic nettle (Urtica dioica) extract on oxidative stress in patients with type 2 diabetes: a randomized double-blind clinical trial. Pak J Biol Sci. 2012 Jan 15;15(2):98-102. PubMed PMID: 22545363

3. Khalili N, Fereydoonzadeh R, Mohtashami R, Mehrzadi S, Heydari M, Huseini HF. Silymarin, Olibanum, and Nettle, A Mixed Herbal Formulation in the Treatment of Type II Diabetes: A Randomized, Double-Blind, Placebo-Controlled, Clinical Trial. J Evid Based Complementary Altern Med. 2017 Oct;22(4):603-608. doi: 10.1177/2156587217696929. Epub 2017 Mar 21. PubMed PMID: 29228792; PubMed Central PMCID: PMC5871270.

Aloe Vera

1. Zhang Y, Liu W, Liu D, Zhao T, Tian H. Efficacy of Aloe Vera Supplementation on Prediabetes and Early Non-Treated Diabetic Patients: A Systematic Review and Meta-Analysis of Randomized Controlled Trials. Nutrients. 2016 Jun 23;8(7). pii: E388. doi: 10.3390/nu8070388. Review. PubMed PMID: 27347994; PubMed Central PMCID: PMC4963864.

2. Choudhary M, Kochhar A, Sangha J. Hypoglycemic and hypolipidemic effect of Aloe vera L. in non-insulin dependent diabetics. J Food Sci Technol. 2014 Jan;51(1):90-6. doi: 10.1007/s13197-011-0459-0. Epub 2011 Jul 16. PubMed PMID: 24426052; PubMed Central PMCID: PMC3857397.

3. Choi HC, Kim SJ, Son KY, Oh BJ, Cho BL. Metabolic effects of aloe vera gel complex in obese prediabetes and early non-treated diabetic patients: randomized controlled trial. Nutrition. 2013 Sep;29(9):1110-4. doi: 10.1016/j.nut.2013.02.015. Epub 2013 Jun 2. PubMed PMID: 23735317.

4. Devaraj S, Yimam M, Brownell LA, Jialal I, Singh S, Jia Q. Effects of Aloe vera supplementation in subjects with prediabetes/metabolic syndrome. Metab Syndr Relat Disord. 2013 Feb;11(1):35-40. doi: 10.1089/met.2012.0066. Epub 2012 Oct 4. PubMed PMID: 23035844.

5. Huseini HF, Kianbakht S, Hajiaghaee R, Dabaghian FH. Anti-hyperglycemic and anti-hypercholesterolemic effects of Aloe vera leaf gel in hyperlipidemic type 2 diabetic patients: a randomized double-blind placebo-controlled clinical trial. Planta Med. 2012 Mar;78(4):311-6. doi: 10.1055/s-0031-1280474. Epub 2011 Dec 23. PubMed PMID: 22198821.

6. Yongchaiyudha S, Rungpitarangsi V, Bunyapraphatsara N, Chokechaijaroenporn O. Antidiabetic activity of Aloe vera L. juice. I. Clinical trial in new cases of diabetes mellitus. Phytomedicine. 1996 Nov;3(3):241-3. doi: 10.1016/S0944-7113(96)80060-2. PubMed PMID: 23195077.

Fig Leaves

1. Mazhin, Sadegh Ahmadi, et al. "Ficus Carica Leaves Decoction on Glycemic Factors of Patients With Type 2 Diabetes Mellitus: A Double-Blind Clinical Trial." Jundishapur Journal of Natural Pharmaceutical Products, vol. 11, no. 1, 2016, doi:10.17795/jjnpp-25814.

Flax Seeds

1. Mani UV, Mani I, Biswas M, Kumar SN. An open-label study on the effect of flax seed powder (Linum usitatissimum) supplementation in the management of diabetes mellitus. J Diet Suppl. 2011 Sep;8(3):257-65. doi: 10.3109/19390211.2011.593615. Epub 2011 Jul 15. PubMed PMID: 22432725.

2. Thakur G, Mitra A, Pal K, Rousseau D. Effect of flaxseed gum on reduction of blood glucose and cholesterol in type 2 diabetic patients. Int J Food Sci Nutr. 2009;60 Suppl 6:126-36. PubMed PMID: 19548163.

Fenugreek

1. Neelakantan N, Narayanan M, de Souza RJ, van Dam RM. Effect of fenugreek (Trigonella foenum-graecum L.) intake on glycemia: a meta-analysis of clinical trials. Nutr J. 2014 Jan 18;13:7. doi: 10.1186/1475-2891-13-7. PubMed PMID: 24438170; PubMed Central PMCID: PMC3901758.

2. Gupta A, Gupta R, Lal B. Effect of Trigonella foenum-graecum (fenugreek) seeds on glycaemic control and insulin resistance in type 2 diabetes mellitus: a double blind placebo controlled study. J Assoc Physicians India. 2001 Nov;49:1057-61. PubMed PMID: 11868855.

3. Bordia A, Verma SK, Srivastava KC. Effect of ginger (Zingiber officinale Rosc.) and fenugreek (Trigonella foenumgraecum L.) on blood lipids, blood sugar and platelet aggregation in patients with coronary artery disease. Prostaglandins Leukot Essent Fatty Acids. 1997 May;56(5):379-84. PubMed PMID: 9175175.

4. Sharma RD, Raghuram TC, Rao NS. Effect of fenugreek seeds on blood glucose and serum lipids in type I diabetes. Eur J Clin Nutr. 1990 Apr;44(4):301-6. PubMed PMID: 2194788.

Caucasian Whortleberry

1. Kianbakht S, Abasi B, Dabaghian FH. Anti-hyperglycemic effect of Vaccinium arctostaphylos in type 2 diabetic patients: a randomized controlled trial. Forsch Komplementmed. 2013;20(1):17-22. doi: 10.1159/000346607. Epub 2013 Feb 19. PubMed PMID: 23727759.

Walnut Leaf

1. Hosseini S, Jamshidi L, Mehrzadi S, Mohammad K, Najmizadeh AR, Alimoradi H, Huseini HF. Effects of Juglans regia L. leaf extract on hyperglycemia and lipid profiles in type two diabetic patients: a randomized double-blind, placebo-controlled clinical trial.J Ethnopharmacol. 2014 Mar 28;152(3):451-6. doi: 10.1016/j.jep.2014.01.012. Epub 2014 Jan 23. PubMed PMID: 24462785.

Jackfruit Leaf (Artocarpus Heterophyllus)

1. G.N, Sree Deepthi, et al. "HYPOGLYCAEMIC EFFECT OF LEAF DECOCTION OF PANASA [ARTOCARPUS HETEROPHYLLUS LAM] IN TYPE II DIABETES MELLITUS- A CLINICAL STUDY." International Journal of Ayurveda and Pharma Research, Oct. 2017, ijapr.in/index.php/ijapr/article/view/807.

Withania Coagulans

1. Upadhyay BN, Gupta V. A clinical study on the effect of Rishyagandha (Withania coagulans) in the management of

Prameha (Type II Diabetes Mellitus). Ayu. 2011 Oct;32(4):507-11. doi: 10.4103/0974-8520.96124. PubMed PMID: 22661845; PubMed Central PMCID: PMC3361926.

Indian Gentian

1. Shankarrao, Yogesh, et al. "CONTROLLED CLINICAL EVALUATION OF MAMAJJAK CHOORNA IN STHULA MADHUMEHA VIZ-A-VIZ TYPE 2 DIABETES MELLITUS." International Journal of Ayurveda and Pharma Research, July 2017, ijapr.in/index.php/ijapr/article/view/715.

2. Kumar S, Singh G, Pandey AK, Singh RH. A clinical study on the Naimittika Rasayana effect of Silajatu and Mamajjaka in type-2 Diabetes Mellitus. Ayu. 2014 Oct-Dec;35(4):404-10. doi: 10.4103/0974-8520.159000. PubMed PMID: 26195903; PubMed Central PMCID: PMC4492025.

American Ginseng

1. Vuksan V, Sievenpiper JL, Wong J, Xu Z, Beljan-Zdravkovic U, Arnason JT, Assinewe V, Stavro MP, Jenkins AL, Leiter LA, Francis T. American ginseng (Panax quinquefolius L.) attenuates postprandial glycemia in a time-dependent but not dose-dependent manner in healthy individuals. Am J Clin Nutr. 2001 Apr;73(4):753-8. PubMed PMID: 11273850.

2. Vuksan V, Stavro MP, Sievenpiper JL, Koo VY, Wong E, Beljan-Zdravkovic U, Francis T, Jenkins AL, Leiter LA, Josse RG, Xu Z. American ginseng improves glycemia in individuals with normal glucose tolerance: effect of dose and time escalation. J Am Coll Nutr. 2000 Nov-Dec;19(6):738-44. PubMed PMID: 11194526.

3. Vuksan V, Stavro MP, Sievenpiper JL, Beljan-Zdravkovic U, Leiter LA, Josse RG, Xu Z. Similar postprandial glycemic reductions with escalation of dose and administration time of American ginseng in type 2 diabetes. Diabetes Care. 2000 Sep;23(9):1221-6. PubMed PMID: 10977009.

4. Vuksan V, Sievenpiper JL, Koo VY, Francis T, Beljan-

Zdravkovic U, Xu Z, Vidgen E. American ginseng (Panax quinquefolius L) reduces postprandial glycemia in nondiabetic subjects and subjects with type 2 diabetes mellitus. Arch Intern Med. 2000 Apr 10;160(7):1009-13. PubMed PMID: 10761967.

Triphala

1. Rajan SS, Antony S. Hypoglycemic effect of triphala on selected non insulin dependent Diabetes mellitus subjects. Anc Sci Life. 2008 Jan;27(3):45-9. PubMed PMID: 22557278; PubMed Central PMCID: PMC3330861.

Shilajit

1. Kumar S, Singh G, Pandey AK, Singh RH. A clinical study on the Naimittika Rasayana effect of Silajatu and Mamajjaka in type-2 Diabetes Mellitus. Ayu. 2014 Oct-Dec;35(4):404-10. doi: 10.4103/0974-8520.159000. PubMed PMID: 26195903; PubMed Central PMCID: PMC4492025.

2. Lamba, Neha, et al. "Clinical Evaluation of Shilajatu in Madhumeha." International Journal of Ayurvedic Medicine, 2015, 6. 24-32. ijam.co.in/index.php/ijam/article/view/06042015.

3. Kaushal, Kumar & Harishankar3 *1Upadhyay, Mishra & K, Avnish. (2009). Effects of combination of Shilajit extract and Ashwagandha (Withania somnifera) on fasting blood sugar and lipid profile. Journal of Pharmacy Research.

4. Gupta V, Keshari BB, Tiwari SK, Murthy KHHVSSN. A comparative study of Shilajatu and Asanadi Ghana Vati in the management of Madhumeha w.s.r. to type-2 diabetes mellitus. Ayu. 2016 Apr-Jun;37(2):120-124. doi: 10.4103/ayu.AYU_211_15. PubMed PMID: 29200750; PubMed Central PMCID: PMC5688834.

Asanadi Ghana Vati

1. Gupta, V & Keshari, B.B. & Tiwari, S.K. & K, Narasimha. (2013). A review on antidiabetic action of asanadi gana. International Journal of Research in Ayurveda and Pharmacy. 4.

638-646. 10.7897/2277_4343.04502.

2. Gupta V, Keshari BB, Tiwari SK, Murthy KHHVSSN. A comparative study of Shilajatu and Asanadi Ghana Vati in the management of Madhumeha w.s.r. to type-2 diabetes mellitus. Ayu. 2016 Apr-Jun;37(2):120-124. doi: 10.4103/ayu.AYU_211_15. PubMed PMID: 29200750; PubMed Central PMCID: PMC5688834.

Ginger

1. Daily, James W., et al. "Efficacy of Ginger for Treating Type 2 Diabetes: A Systematic Review and Meta-Analysis of Randomized Clinical Trials." Journal of Ethnic Foods, vol. 2, no. 1, 2015, pp. 36–43., doi:10.1016/j.jef.2015.02.007.

Garlic

1. Wang J, Zhang X, Lan H, Wang W. Effect of garlic supplement in the management of type 2 diabetes mellitus (T2DM): a meta-analysis of randomized controlled trials. Food Nutr Res. 2017 Sep 27;61(1):1377571. doi: 10.1080/16546628.2017.1377571. eCollection 2017. PubMed PMID: 29056888; PubMed Central PMCID: PMC5642189.

Mehamudgara

1. Tanna I, Chandola HM, Joshi JR. Clinical efficacy of Mehamudgara vati in type 2 diabetes mellitus. Ayu. 2011 Jan;32(1):30-9. doi: 10.4103/0974-8520.85722. PubMed PMID: 22131755; PubMed Central PMCID: PMC3215414.

Phalatrikadi Kwath

1. Jena, Sonalika, et al. "A COMPARATIVE PLACEBO, CONTROL CLINICAL EVALUATION OF PHALATRIKADI KWATH IN MADHUMEHA WITH SPECIAL REFERENCE TO DIABETES MELLITUS TYPE2." International Journal of Ayurveda and Pharma Research, Oct. 2015,

Caper Bush Fruit

1. Huseini HF, Hasani-Rnjbar S, Nayebi N, Heshmat R, Sigaroodi FK, Ahvazi M, Alaei BA, Kianbakht S. Capparis spinosa L. (Caper) fruit extract in treatment of type 2 diabetic patients: a randomized double-blind placebo-controlled clinical trial. Complement Ther Med. 2013 Oct;21(5):447-52. doi: 10.1016/j.ctim.2013.07.003. Epub 2013 Aug 7. PubMed PMID: 24050578.

Bitter Apple

1. Barghamdi B, Ghorat F, Asadollahi K, Sayehmiri K, Peyghambari R, Abangah G. Therapeutic effects of Citrullus colocynthis fruit in patients with type II diabetes: A clinical trial study. J Pharm Bioallied Sci. 2016 Apr-Jun;8(2):130-4. doi: 10.4103/0975-7406.171702. PubMed PMID: 27134465; PubMed Central PMCID: PMC4832903.

2. Huseini HF, Darvishzadeh F, Heshmat R, Jafariazar Z, Raza M, Larijani B. The clinical investigation of Citrullus colocynthis (L.) schrad fruit in treatment of Type II diabetic patients: a randomized, double blind, placebo-controlled clinical trial. Phytother Res. 2009 Aug;23(8):1186-9. doi: 10.1002/ptr.2754. PubMed PMID: 19170143.

Milk Thistle

1. Huseini HF, Larijani B, Heshmat R, Fakhrzadeh H, Radjabipour B, Toliat T, Raza M. The efficacy of Silybum marianum (L.) Gaertn. (silymarin) in the treatment of type II diabetes: a randomized, double-blind, placebo-controlled, clinical trial. Phytother Res. 2006 Dec;20(12):1036-9. PubMed PMID: 17072885.

2. Khalili N, Fereydoonzadeh R, Mohtashami R, Mehrzadi S, Heydari M, Huseini HF. Silymarin, Olibanum, and Nettle, A Mixed Herbal Formulation in the Treatment of Type II Diabetes: A Randomized, Double-Blind, Placebo-Controlled, Clinical Trial. J Evid Based Complementary Altern Med. 2017 Oct;22(4):603-608. doi: 10.1177/2156587217696929. Epub 2017 Mar 21. PubMed PMID: 29228792; PubMed Central PMCID: PMC5871270.

Diabetic Complications

Neuropathy

Bitter Melon

1. Heydari M, Homayouni K, Hashempur MH, Shams M. Topical Citrullus colocynthis (bitter apple) extract oil in painful diabetic neuropathy: A double-blind randomized placebo-controlled clinical trial. J Diabetes. 2016 Mar;8(2):246-52. doi: 10.1111/1753-0407.12287. Epub 2015 Jun 29. PubMed PMID: 25800045.

Guduchyadi Kwath

1. Rehana, Parveen, and B P Sarma. "A Clinical Study To Evaluate The Efficacy Of Guduchyadi Kwath In The Management Of Diabetic Polyneuropathy." International Journal of Research in Ayurveda & Pharmacy, vol. 7, no. 2, 2016, pp. 17–22., doi:10.7897/2277-4343.07248.

Atibalamula & Bhumyamalaki

1. Patel K, Patel M, Gupta SN. Effect of Atibalamula and Bhumyamalaki on thirty-three patients of diabetic neuropathy. Ayu. 2011 Jul;32(3):353-6. doi: 10.4103/0974-8520.93913. PubMed PMID: 22529650; PubMed Central PMCID: PMC3326881.

ALA

1. Reljanovic M, Reichel G, Rett K, Lobisch M, Schuette K, Möller W, Tritschler HJ, Mehnert H. Treatment of diabetic polyneuropathy with the antioxidant thioctic acid (alpha-lipoic acid): a two year multicenter randomized double-blind placebo-controlled trial (ALADIN II). Alpha Lipoic Acid in Diabetic Neuropathy. Free Radic Res. 1999 Sep;31(3):171-9. PubMed PMID: 10499773

Benfotiamine

1. Haupt E, Ledermann H, Köpcke W. Benfotiamine in the treatment of diabetic polyneuropathy--a three-week randomized, controlled pilot study (BEDIP study). Int J Clin Pharmacol Ther. 2005 Feb;43(2):71-7. Erratum in: Int J Clin Pharmacol Ther. 2005 Jun;43(6):304. PubMed PMID: 15726875.

2. Winkler G, Pál B, Nagybéganyi E, Ory I, Porochnavec M, Kempler P. Effectiveness of different benfotiamine dosage regimens in the treatment of painful diabetic neuropathy. Arzneimittelforschung. 1999 Mar;49(3):220-4. PubMed PMID: 10219465.

3. Stracke H, Lindemann A, Federlin K. A benfotiamine-vitamin B combination in treatment of diabetic polyneuropathy. Exp Clin Endocrinol Diabetes. 1996;104(4):311-6. PubMed PMID: 8886748.

Micronutrients (Zinc, Vitamins C, E, B1, B2, B6, B12, Biotin, Folic Acid, Magnesium)

1. Farvid MS, Homayouni F, Amiri Z, Adelmanesh F. Improving neuropathy scores in type 2 diabetic patients using micronutrients supplementation. Diabetes Res Clin Pract. 2011 Jul;93(1):86-94. doi: 10.1016/j.diabres.2011.03.016. Epub 2011 Apr 14. PubMed PMID: 21496936.

Nephropathy

Trypterygium Woldordii

1. Ge Y, Xie H, Li S, Jin B, Hou J, Zhang H, Shi M, Liu Z. Treatment of diabetic nephropathy with Tripterygium wilfordii Hook F extract: a prospective, randomized, controlled clinical trial. J Transl Med. 2013 May 31;11:134. doi: 10.1186/1479-5876-11-134. PubMed PMID: 23725518; PubMed Central PMCID: PMC3670993.

Ginkgo Biloba

1. Zhang L, Mao W, Guo X, Wu Y, Li C, Lu Z, Su G, Li X, Liu Z, Guo R, Jie X, Wen Z, Liu X. Ginkgo biloba Extract for Patients

with Early Diabetic Nephropathy: A Systematic Review. Evid Based Complement Alternat Med. 2013;2013:689142. doi: 10.1155/2013/689142. Epub 2013 Feb 24. PubMed PMID: 23533513; PubMed Central PMCID: PMC3595672.

Silymarin

1. Fallahzadeh MK, Dormanesh B, Sagheb MM, Roozbeh J, Vessal G, Pakfetrat M, Daneshbod Y, Kamali-Sarvestani E, Lankarani KB. Effect of addition of silymarin to renin-angiotensin system inhibitors on proteinuria in type 2 diabetic patients with overt nephropathy: a randomized, double-blind, placebo-controlled trial. Am J Kidney Dis. 2012 Dec;60(6):896-903. doi: 10.1053/j.ajkd.2012.06.005. Epub 2012 Jul 7. PubMed PMID: 22770926

Ayurvedic Protocols

1. Akarshini AM, Aruna. Management of Madhumeha Janya Upadrava with special reference to diabetic nephropathy - A clinical study. Ayu. 2014 Oct-Dec;35(4):378-83. doi: 10.4103/0974-8520.158987. PubMed PMID: 26195899; PubMed Central PMCID: PMC4492021.

2. Patel K, Gupta SN, Shah N. Effect of Ayurvedic management in 130 patients of diabetic nephropathy. Ayu. 2011 Jan;32(1):55-8. doi: 10.4103/0974-8520.85727. PubMed PMID: 22131758; PubMed Central PMCID: PMC3215418.

<u>Retinopathy</u>

Triphala

1. Vd. Sampat, Bhatane G. "EFFECT OF TRIPHALA GHRITA NETRATARPANA IN DIABETIC RETINOPATHY ." International Ayurvedic Medical Journal, vol. 4, no. 8, Aug. 2016, www.iamj.in/posts/images/upload/2519_2521.pdf.

<u>Non-Healing Wounds</u>

Neem Oil & Turmeric

1. Singh A, Singh AK, Narayan G, Singh TB, Shukla VK. Effect of Neem oil and Haridra on non-healing wounds. Ayu. 2014 Oct-Dec;35(4):398-403. doi: 10.4103/0974-8520.158998. PubMed PMID: 26195902; PubMed Central PMCID: PMC4492024.

Manuka Honey

2. Kamaratos AV, Tzirogiannis KN, Iraklianou SA, Panoutsopoulos GI, Kanellos IE, Melidonis AI. Manuka honey-impregnated dressings in the treatment of neuropathic diabetic foot ulcers. Int Wound J. 2014 Jun;11(3):259-63. doi: 10.1111/j.1742-481X.2012.01082.x. Epub 2012 Sep 18. PubMed PMID: 22985336.

Diabetic Nutrition

Chromium

1. Jamilian M, Asemi Z. Chromium Supplementation and the Effects on Metabolic Status in Women with Polycystic Ovary Syndrome: A Randomized, Double-Blind, Placebo-Controlled Trial. Ann Nutr Metab. 2015;67(1):42-8. PubMed PMID: 26279073.

2. Kim CW, Kim BT, Park KH, Kim KM, Lee DJ, Yang SW, Joo NS. Effects of short-term chromium supplementation on insulin sensitivity and body composition in overweight children: randomized, double-blind, placebo-controlled study. J Nutr Biochem. 2011 Nov;22(11):1030-4. doi: 10.1016/j.jnutbio.2010.10.001. Epub 2011 Jan 8. PubMed PMID: 21216583.

3. Aghdassi E, Arendt BM, Salit IE, Mohammed SS, Jalali P, Bondar H, Allard JP. In patients with HIV-infection, chromium supplementation improves insulin resistance and other metabolic abnormalities: a randomized, double-blind, placebo controlled trial. Curr HIV Res. 2010 Mar;8(2):113-20. PubMed PMID: 20163347.

4. Anderson RA. Chromium and polyphenols from cinnamon improve insulin sensitivity. Proc Nutr Soc. 2008 Feb;67(1):48-53.

doi: 10.1017/S0029665108006010. PubMed PMID: 18234131.

5. Preuss HG, Bagchi D, Bagchi M, Rao CV, Dey DK, Satyanarayana S. Effects of a natural extract of (-)-hydroxycitric acid (HCA-SX) and a combination of HCA-SX plus niacin-bound chromium and Gymnema sylvestre extract on weight loss. Diabetes Obes Metab. 2004 May;6(3):171-80. PubMed PMID: 15056124.

6. A scientific review: the role of chromium in insulin resistance. Diabetes Educ. 2004;Suppl:2-14. Review. PubMed PMID: 15208835

7. Ghosh D, Bhattacharya B, Mukherjee B, Manna B, Sinha M, Chowdhury J, Chowdhury S. Role of chromium supplementation in Indians with type 2 diabetes mellitus. J Nutr Biochem. 2002 Nov;13(11):690-697. PubMed PMID: 12550067.

Vanadium

1. Cusi K, Cukier S, DeFronzo RA, Torres M, Puchulu FM, Redondo JC. Vanadyl sulfate improves hepatic and muscle insulin sensitivity in type 2 diabetes. J Clin Endocrinol Metab. 2001 Mar;86(3):1410-7. PubMed PMID: 11238540.

2. Halberstam M, Cohen N, Shlimovich P, Rossetti L, Shamoon H. Oral vanadyl sulfate improves insulin sensitivity in NIDDM but not in obese nondiabetic subjects. Diabetes. 1996 May;45(5):659-66. Erratum in: Diabetes 1996 Sep;45(9):1285. PubMed PMID: 8621019.

3. Cohen N, Halberstam M, Shlimovich P, Chang CJ, Shamoon H, Rossetti L. Oral vanadyl sulfate improves hepatic and peripheral insulin sensitivity in patients with non-insulin-dependent diabetes mellitus. J Clin Invest. 1995 Jun;95(6):2501-9. PubMed PMID: 7769096; PubMed Central PMCID: PMC295932.

Benfotiamine

1. Beltramo E, Berrone E, Tarallo S, Porta M. Effects of thiamine and benfotiamine on intracellular glucose metabolism and

relevance in the prevention of diabetic complications. Acta Diabetol. 2008 Sep;45(3):131-41. doi: 10.1007/s00592-008-0042-y. Epub 2008 Jun 26. Review. PubMed PMID: 18581039.

2. Berrone E, Beltramo E, Solimine C, Ape AU, Porta M. Regulation of intracellular glucose and polyol pathway by thiamine and benfotiamine in vascular cells cultured in high glucose. J Biol Chem. 2006 Apr 7;281(14):9307-13. Epub 2006 Feb 1. PubMed PMID: 16452468

Magnesium

1. Simental-Mendía LE, Sahebkar A, Rodríguez-Morán M, Guerrero-Romero F. A systematic review and meta-analysis of randomized controlled trials on the effects of magnesium supplementation on insulin sensitivity and glucose control. Pharmacol Res. 2016 Sep;111:272-282. doi: 10.1016/j.phrs.2016.06.019. Epub 2016 Jun 18. Review. PubMed PMID: 27329332

2. Solati M, Ouspid E, Hosseini S, Soltani N, Keshavarz M, Dehghani M. Oral magnesium supplementation in type II diabetic patients.Med J Islam Repub Iran. 2014 Jul 15;28:67. eCollection 2014. PubMed PMID: 25405132; PubMed Central PMCID: PMC4219896.

3. De Leeuw I, Engelen W, De Block C, Van Gaal L. Long term magnesium supplementation influences favourably the natural evolution of neuropathy in Mg-depleted type 1 diabetic patients (T1dm). Magnes Res. 2004 Jun;17(2):109-14. PubMed PMID: 15319143.

4. Rodríguez-Morán M, Guerrero-Romero F. Oral magnesium supplementation improves insulin sensitivity and metabolic control in type 2 diabetic subjects: a randomized double-blind controlled trial. Diabetes Care. 2003 Apr;26(4):1147-52. PubMed PMID: 12663588

Vitamin A

1. Yosaee S, Akbari Fakhrabadi M, Shidfar F. Positive evidence

for vitamin A role in prevention of type 1 diabetes. World J Diabetes. 2016 May 10;7(9):177-88. doi: 10.4239/wjd.v7.i9.177. Review. PubMed PMID: 27162582; PubMed Central PMCID: PMC4856890.

Exercise, Yoga & Diet

Exercise

1. Stanford KI, Goodyear LJ. Exercise and type 2 diabetes: molecular mechanisms regulating glucose uptake in skeletal muscle. Adv Physiol Educ. 2014 Dec;38(4):308-14. doi: 10.1152/advan.00080.2014. Review. PubMed PMID: 25434013; PubMed Central PMCID: PMC4315445.

2. Colberg SR, Sigal RJ, Fernhall B, Regensteiner JG, Blissmer BJ, Rubin RR, Chasan-Taber L, Albright AL, Braun B; American College of Sports Medicine.; American Diabetes Association.. Exercise and type 2 diabetes: the American College of Sports Medicine and the American Diabetes Association: joint position statement. Diabetes Care. 2010 Dec;33(12):e147-67. doi: 10.2337/dc10-9990. PubMed PMID: 21115758; PubMed Central PMCID: PMC2992225.

3. Richter EA, Derave W, Wojtaszewski JF. Glucose, exercise and insulin: emerging concepts. J Physiol. 2001 Sep 1;535(Pt 2):313-22. Review. PubMed PMID: 11533125; PubMed Central PMCID: PMC2278791.

4. Kennedy JW, Hirshman MF, Gervino EV, Ocel JV, Forse RA, Hoenig SJ, Aronson D, Goodyear LJ, Horton ES. Acute exercise induces GLUT4 translocation in skeletal muscle of normal human subjects and subjects with type 2 diabetes. Diabetes. 1999 May;48(5):1192-7. PubMed PMID: 10331428.

Yoga

1. Jayawardena R, Ranasinghe P, Chathuranga T, Atapattu PM, Misra A. The benefits of yoga practice compared to physical exercise in the management of type 2 Diabetes Mellitus: A systematic review and meta-analysis. Diabetes Metab Syndr. 2018

Apr 18. pii: S1871-4021(18)30090-0. doi: 10.1016/j.dsx.2018.04.008. [Epub ahead of print] Review. PubMed PMID: 29685823.

2. Cui J, Yan JH, Yan LM, Pan L, Le JJ, Guo YZ. Effects of yoga in adults with type 2 diabetes mellitus: A meta-analysis. J Diabetes Investig. 2017 Mar;8(2):201-209. doi: 10.1111/jdi.12548. Epub 2016 Sep 19. PubMed PMID: 27370357; PubMed Central PMCID: PMC5334310.

3. Vinutha HT, Raghavendra BR, Manjunath NK. Effect of integrated approach of yoga therapy on autonomic functions in patients with type 2 diabetes. Indian J Endocrinol Metab. 2015 Sep-Oct;19(5):653-7. doi: 10.4103/2230-8210.163194. PubMed PMID: 26425477; PubMed Central PMCID: PMC4566348.

4. Chimkode SM, Kumaran SD, Kanhere VV, Shivanna R. Effect of yoga on blood glucose levels in patients with type 2 diabetes mellitus. J Clin Diagn Res. 2015 Apr;9(4):CC01-3. doi: 10.7860/JCDR/2015/12666.5744. Epub 2015 Apr 1. PubMed PMID: 26023550; PubMed Central PMCID: PMC4437062.

5. Singh S, Kyizom T, Singh KP, Tandon OP, Madhu SV. Influence of pranayamas and yoga-asanas on serum insulin, blood glucose and lipid profile in type 2 diabetes. Indian J Clin Biochem. 2008 Oct;23(4):365-8. doi: 10.1007/s12291-008-0080-9. Epub 2008 Dec 20. PubMed PMID: 23105788; PubMed Central PMCID: PMC3453135.

Diet

1. Hussain TA, Mathew TC, Dashti AA, Asfar S, Al-Zaid N, Dashti HM. Effect of low-calorie versus low-carbohydrate ketogenic diet in type 2 diabetes. Nutrition. 2012 Oct;28(10):1016-21. doi: 10.1016/j.nut.2012.01.016. Epub 2012 Jun 5. PubMed PMID: 22673594.

2. Westman EC, Yancy WS Jr, Mavropoulos JC, Marquart M, McDuffie JR.The effect of a low-carbohydrate, ketogenic diet versus a low-glycemic index diet on glycemic control in type 2 diabetes mellitus.Nutr Metab (Lond). 2008 Dec 19;5:36. doi:

10.1186/1743-7075-5-36. PubMed PMID: 19099589; PubMed Central PMCID: PMC2633336.

3. Yancy WS Jr, Foy M, Chalecki AM, Vernon MC, Westman EC. A low-carbohydrate, ketogenic diet to treat type 2 diabetes. Nutr Metab (Lond). 2005 Dec 1;2:34. PubMed PMID: 16318637; PubMed Central PMCID: PMC1325029.

Diabetes Type 1

1. Shanmugasundaram ER, Rajeswari G, Baskaran K, Rajesh Kumar BR, Radha Shanmugasundaram K, Kizar Ahmath B. Use of Gymnema sylvestre leaf extract in the control of blood glucose in insulin-dependent diabetes mellitus. J Ethnopharmacol. 1990 Oct;30(3):281-94. PubMed PMID: 2259216

2. Baldwa VS, Bhandari CM, Pangaria A, Goyal RK. Clinical trial in patients with diabetes mellitus of an insulin-like compound obtained from plant source. Ups J Med Sci. 1977;82(1):39-41. doi: 10.3109/03009737709179057. PubMed PMID: 20078273.

3. Ahmad N, Hassan MR, Halder H, Bennoor KS. Effect of Momordica charantia (Karolla) extracts on fasting and postprandial serum glucose levels in NIDDM patients. Bangladesh Med Res Counc Bull. 1999 Apr;25(1):11-3. PubMed PMID: 10758656.

4. Sharma RD, Raghuram TC, Rao NS. Effect of fenugreek seeds on blood glucose and serum lipids in type I diabetes. Eur J Clin Nutr. 1990 Apr;44(4):301-6. PubMed PMID: 2194788.

Additional References related to Mode of action

Amla

1. K.V.Santhi Sri, et al. "Effect of Amla, an Approach towards the Control of Diabetes Mellitus." *International Journal of Current Microbiology and Applied Sciences*, vol. 2, no. 9, 2013, pp. 103–108., www.ijcmas.com/vol-2-9/K.V.Santhi Sri, et al.pdf.

2. To cite this article: Shikha Mehta, Rakesh Kumar Singh, Dolly Jaiswal, Prashant Kumar Rai & Geeta Watal (2009) Anti-diabetic activity of Emblicaofficinalis in animal models, Pharmaceutical Biology, 47:11, 1050-1055, DOI: 10.3109/13880200902991532

3. K. Walia, and R. Boolchandani. "Role of Amla in Type 2 Diabetes Mellitus - A Review." *Research Journal of Recent Sciences*, vol. 4, no. (ISC-2014), 2015, pp. 31–35., www.isca.in/rjrs/archive/v4/iISC-2014/8.ISCA-ISC-2014-Poster-13PCS-09.pdf.

Berberine

1. Yin, Jun, et al. "Effects and Mechanisms of Berberine in Diabetes Treatment." *Acta Pharmaceutica Sinica B*, vol. 2, no. 4, 2012, pp. 327–334., doi:https://doi.org/10.1016/j.apsb.2012.06.003.

Nettle

1. Hailemeskel, Bisrat & Fullas, Fekadu. (2016). The Use of Urtica dioica (Stinging Nettle) as a Blood Sugar Lowering Herb: A Case Report and a Review of the Literature. Diabetes Research - Open Journal. 1. 123-127. 10.17140/DROJ-1-119.

2. Gohari A, Noorafshan A, Akmali M, Zamani-Garmsiri F, Seghatoleslam A. Urtica Dioica Distillate Regenerates Pancreatic Beta Cells in Streptozotocin-Induced Diabetic Rats. Iran J Med Sci. 2018 Mar;43(2):174-183. PubMed PMID: 29749986; PubMed Central PMCID: PMC5936849.

3. Qujeq D, Tatar M, Feizi F, Parsian H, Sohan Faraji A, Halalkhor S. Effect of Urtica dioica Leaf Alcoholic and Aqueous Extracts on the Number and the Diameter of the Islets in Diabetic Rats. Int J Mol Cell Med. 2013 Winter;2(1):21-6. PubMed PMID: 24551786; PubMed Central PMCID: PMC3920518.

Ficus Carica

1. Ramgopal Mopuri, Muniswamy Ganjayi, Balaji Meriga, Neil Anthony Koorbanally, Md. Shahidul Islam, The effects of Ficus

carica on the activity of enzymes related to metabolic syndrome, Journal of Food and Drug Analysis, Volume 26, Issue 1, 2018, Pages 201-210, ISSN 1021-9498, https://doi.org/10.1016/j.jfda.2017.03.001 (http://www.sciencedirect.com/science/article/pii/S1021949817300765)

2. Pérez C, Domínguez E, Canal JR, Campillo JE, Torres MD. Hypoglycaemic activity of an aqueous extract from ficus carica (fig tree) leaves in streptozotocin diabetic rats. Pharm Biol. 2000;38(3):181-6. doi: 10.1076/1388-0209(200007)3831-SFT181. PubMed PMID: 21214459.

3. Stephen Irudayaraj S, Christudas S, Antony S, Duraipandiyan V, Naif Abdullah AD, Ignacimuthu S. Protective effects of Ficus carica leaves on glucose and lipids levels, carbohydrate metabolism enzymes and β-cells in type 2 diabetic rats. Pharm Biol. 2017 Dec;55(1):1074-1081. doi: 10.1080/13880209.2017.1279671. PubMed PMID: 28193094; PubMed Central PMCID: PMC6130661.

Flax Seed

1. Kshitij Bhardwaj, Narsingh Verma, R.K. Trivedi and Shipra Bhardwaj, 2015. Flaxseed Oil and Diabetes: A Systemic Review. *Journal of Medical Sciences, 15: 135-138.* DOI:10.3923/jms.2015.135.138. https://scialert.net/abstract/?doi=jms.2015.135.138

2. Prasad K, Dhar A. Flaxseed and Diabetes. Curr Pharm Des. 2016;22(2):141-4. Review. PubMed PMID: 26561065.

3. Dusane MB, Joshi BN. Beneficial effect of flax seeds in streptozotocin (STZ) induced diabetic mice: isolation of active fraction having islet regenerative and glucosidase inhibitory properties. Can J Physiol Pharmacol. 2013 May;91(5):325-31. doi: 10.1139/cjpp-2011-0428. Epub 2013 Jan 16. PubMed PMID: 23656171.

Fenugreek

1. K. Srinivasan (2006) Fenugreek (*Trigonella foenum-graecum*): A Review of Health Beneficial Physiological Effects, Food Reviews International, 22:2, 203-224, DOI: 10.1080/87559120600586315

2. Xue WL, Li XS, Zhang J, Liu YH, Wang ZL, Zhang RJ. Effect of Trigonella foenum-graecum (fenugreek) extract on blood glucose, blood lipid and hemorheological properties in streptozotocin-induced diabetic rats. Asia Pac J Clin Nutr. 2007;16 Suppl 1:422-6. PubMed PMID: 17392143.

Caucasian Whortleberry

1. Firouzeh M, Shahanipour K. The effects of Vaccinium arctostaphylos L. extract on the levels of glucose, oxidation indicators, HDL and cholesterol in diabetic rats (Wistar).. jmj. 2015; 13 (4) :23-32
URL: http://jmj.jums.ac.ir/article-1-581-en.html

2. Kianbakht S, Hajiaghaee R. Anti-hyperglycemic Effects of Vaccinium arctostaphylos L. Fruit and Leaf Extracts in Alloxan-Induced Diabetic Rats. JMP. 2013; 1 (45) :43-50
URL: http://jmp.ir/article-1-108-en.html

Shilajit

1. Trivedi N A, Mazumdar B, Bhatt J D, Hemavathi K G. Effect of shilajit on blood glucose and lipid profile in alloxan-induced diabetic rats. Indian J Pharmacol 2004;36:373-6

Bitter Apple

1. Esmaeel Ebrahimi, Somaieh Bahramzadeh, Mahmoud Hashemitabar, Ghorban Mohammadzadeh, Saeed Shirali, Javad Jodat, Effect of hydroalcoholic leaves extract of Citrullus colocynthis on induction of insulin secretion from isolated rat islets of Langerhans, Asian Pacific Journal of Tropical Disease, Volume 6, Issue 8, 2016, Pages 638-641, ISSN 2222-1808, https://doi.org/10.1016/S2222-1808(16)61101-5.

(http://www.sciencedirect.com/science/article/pii/S2222180816611015)

2. Selvaraj, Gurudeeban & Kaliamurthi, Satyavani &, Ramanathan. (2012). Alpha glucosidase inhibitory effect and enzyme kinetics of coastal medicinal plants. Bangladesh Journal of Pharmacology. 7. 186-191. 10.3329/bjp.v7i3.11499.

3. Benariba N, Djaziri R, Hupkens E, Louchami K, Malaisse WJ, Sener A. Insulinotropic action of Citrullus colocynthis seed extracts in rat pancreatic islets. Mol Med Rep. 2013 Jan;7(1):233-6. doi: 10.3892/mmr.2012.1151. Epub 2012 Oct 24. PubMed PMID: 23128986

4. Nmila R, Gross R, Rchid H, Roye M, Manteghetti M, Petit P, Tijane M, Ribes G, Sauvaire Y. Insulinotropic effect of Citrullus colocynthis fruit extracts. Planta Med. 2000 Jun;66(5):418-23. PubMed PMID: 10909260.

Ginger

1. James W. Daily, Mini Yang, Da Sol Kim, Sunmin Park, Efficacy of ginger for treating Type 2 diabetes: A systematic review and meta-analysis of randomized clinical trials, Journal of Ethnic Foods, Volume 2, Issue 1, 2015, Pages 36-43, ISSN 2352-6181, https://doi.org/10.1016/j.jef.2015.02.007 (http://www.sciencedirect.com/science/article/pii/S2352618115000086)

Sage

1. Hamidpour M, Hamidpour R, Hamidpour S, Shahlari M. Chemistry, Pharmacology, and Medicinal Property of Sage (Salvia) to Prevent and Cure Illnesses such as Obesity, Diabetes, Depression, Dementia, Lupus, Autism, Heart Disease, and Cancer. J Tradit Complement Med. 2014 Apr;4(2):82-8. doi: 10.4103/2225-4110.130373. Review. PubMed PMID: 24860730; PubMed Central PMCID: PMC4003706.

2. Lima CF, Azevedo MF, Araujo R, Fernandes-Ferreira M, Pereira-Wilson C. Metformin-like effect of Salvia officinalis

(common sage): is it useful in diabetes prevention? Br J Nutr. 2006 Aug;96(2):326-33. PubMed PMID: 16923227.

Aloe

1. Yimam M, Zhao J, Corneliusen B, Pantier M, Brownell L, Jia Q. Blood glucose lowering activity of aloe based composition, UP780, in alloxan induced insulin dependent mouse diabetes model. Diabetol Metab Syndr. 2014 May 24;6:61. doi: 10.1186/1758-5996-6-61. eCollection 2014. PubMed PMID: 24891878; PubMed Central PMCID: PMC4041641

2. Ajabnoor MA. Effect of aloes on blood glucose levels in normal and alloxan diabetic mice. J Ethnopharmacol. 1990 Feb;28(2):215-20. PubMed PMID: 2109811.

Nigella Sativa

1. Kaatabi H, Bamosa AO, Badar A, Al-Elq A, Abou-Hozaifa B, Lebda F, Al-Khadra A, Al-Almaie S. Nigella sativa improves glycemic control and ameliorates oxidative stress in patients with type 2 diabetes mellitus: placebo controlled participant blinded clinical trial. PLoS One. 2015 Feb 23;10(2):e0113486. doi: 10.1371/journal.pone.0113486. eCollection 2015. PubMed PMID: 25706772; PubMed Central PMCID: PMC4338020.

2. Benhaddou-Andaloussi A, Martineau L, Vuong T, Meddah B, Madiraju P, Settaf A, Haddad PS. The In Vivo Antidiabetic Activity of Nigella sativa Is Mediated through Activation of the AMPK Pathway and Increased Muscle Glut4 Content. Evid Based Complement Alternat Med. 2011;2011:538671. doi: 10.1155/2011/538671. Epub 2011 Apr 14. PubMed PMID: 21584245; PubMed Central PMCID: PMC3092603.

3. Fararh KM, Atoji Y, Shimizu Y, Shiina T, Nikami H, Takewaki T. Mechanisms of the hypoglycaemic and immunopotentiating effects of Nigella sativa L. oil in streptozotocin-induced diabetic hamsters. Res Vet Sci. 2004 Oct;77(2):123-9. PubMed PMID: 15196902.

Indian Gentian

1. Maroo J, Vasu VT, Aalinkeel R, Gupta S. Glucose lowering effect of aqueous extract of Enicostemma littorale Blume in diabetes: a possible mechanism of action. J Ethnopharmacol. 2002 Aug;81(3):317-20. PubMed PMID: 12127231.

Withania Coagulans

1. Shukla K, Dikshit P, Shukla R, Gambhir JK. The aqueous extract of Withania coagulans fruit partially reverses nicotinamide/streptozotocin-induced diabetes mellitus in rats. J Med Food. 2012 Aug;15(8):718-25. doi: 10.1089/jmf.2011.1829. Epub 2012 Jun 25. PubMed PMID: 22846078; PubMed Central PMCID: PMC3407382.

Walnut Leaf

1. Javidanpour S, Fatemi Tabtabaei SR, Siahpoosh A, Morovati H, Shahriari A. Comparison of the effects of fresh leaf and peel extracts of walnut (Juglans regia L.) on blood glucose and β-cells of streptozotocin-induced diabetic rats. Vet Res Forum. 2012 Fall;3(4):251-5. PubMed PMID: 25653767; PubMed Central PMCID: PMC4313044.

2. Nasiry D, Khalatbary AR, Ahmadvand H, Talebpour Amiri F, Akbari E. Protective effects of methanolic extract of Juglans regia L. leaf on streptozotocin-induced diabetic peripheral neuropathy in rats. BMC Complement Altern Med. 2017 Oct 2;17(1):476. doi: 10.1186/s12906-017-1983-x. PubMed PMID: 28969623; PubMed Central PMCID: PMC5625610.

Caper Fruit

1. Zhang H, Ma ZF. Phytochemical and Pharmacological Properties of Capparis spinosa as a Medicinal Plant. Nutrients. 2018 Jan 24;10(2). pii: E116. doi: 10.3390/nu10020116. Review. PubMed PMID: 29364841; PubMed Central PMCID: PMC5852692.

2. Vahid H, Rakhshandeh H, Ghorbani A. Antidiabetic properties

of Capparis spinosa L. and its components. Biomed Pharmacother. 2017 Aug;92:293-302. doi: 10.1016/j.biopha.2017.05.082. Review. PubMed PMID: 28551550.

3. Kazemian M, Abad M, Haeri MR, Ebrahimi M, Heidari R. Antidiabetic effect of Capparis spinosa L. root extract in diabetic rats. Avicenna J Phytomed. 2015 Jul-Aug;5(4):325-32. PubMed PMID: 26445712; PubMed Central PMCID: PMC4587611.

Triphala

1. Peterson CT, Denniston K, Chopra D. Therapeutic Uses of Triphala in Ayurvedic Medicine. J Altern Complement Med. 2017 Aug;23(8):607-614. doi: 10.1089/acm.2017.0083. Epub 2017 Jul 11. Review. PubMed PMID: 28696777; PubMed Central PMCID: PMC5567597.

Cinnamon

1. Medagama AB. The glycaemic outcomes of Cinnamon, a review of the experimental evidence and clinical trials. Nutr J. 2015 Oct 16;14:108. doi: 10.1186/s12937-015-0098-9. Review. PubMed PMID: 26475130; PubMed Central PMCID: PMC4609100.

Vinegar

1. Mitrou P, Petsiou E, Papakonstantinou E, Maratou E, Lambadiari V, Dimitriadis P, Spanoudi F, Raptis SA, Dimitriadis G. Vinegar Consumption Increases Insulin-Stimulated Glucose Uptake by the Forearm Muscle in Humans with Type 2 Diabetes. J Diabetes Res. 2015;2015:175204. doi: 10.1155/2015/175204. Epub 2015 May 6. PubMed PMID: 26064976; PubMed Central PMCID: PMC4438142.

Garlic

1. Liu CT, Hsu TW, Chen KM, Tan YP, Lii CK, Sheen LY. The Antidiabetic Effect of Garlic Oil is Associated with Ameliorated Oxidative Stress but Not Ameliorated Level of Pro-inflammatory Cytokines in Skeletal Muscle of Streptozotocin-induced Diabetic

Rats. J Tradit Complement Med. 2012 Apr;2(2):135-44. PubMed PMID: 24716126; PubMed Central PMCID: PMC3942916.

Jackfruit Leaf

1. Chackrewarthy S, Thabrew MI, Weerasuriya MK, Jayasekera S. Evaluation of the hypoglycemic and hypolipidemic effects of an ethylacetate fraction of Artocarpus heterophyllus (jak) leaves in streptozotocin-induced diabetic rats. Pharmacogn Mag. 2010 Jul;6(23):186-90. doi: 10.4103/0973-1296.66933. PubMed PMID: 20931077; PubMed Central PMCID: PMC2950380

Ginseng

1. Luo JZ, Luo L. Ginseng on hyperglycemia: effects and mechanisms. Evid Based Complement Alternat Med. 2009 Dec;6(4):423-7. doi: 10.1093/ecam/nem178. Epub 2008 Jan 3. PubMed PMID: 18955300; PubMed Central PMCID: PMC2781779.

Milk Thistle

1. Kazazis CE, Evangelopoulos AA, Kollas A, Vallianou NG. The therapeutic potential of milk thistle in diabetes. Rev Diabet Stud. 2014 Summer;11(2):167-74. doi: 10.1900/RDS.2014.11.167. Epub 2014 Aug 10. Review. PubMed PMID: 25396404; PubMed Central PMCID: PMC4310066

www.ingramcontent.com/pod-product-compliance
Lightning Source LLC
Chambersburg PA
CBHW071536220526
45469CB00003B/802